Tradepaper ISBN 978-1-5272-8007-6

First printed edition, April 2021 in UK

Publisher
BRAHMANI YOGA
www.brahmaniyoga.com

Editor: Jodi Marcus
Project managers: Myrthe Wieler & Deborah Rossi
Design and layout: Bjarney Hinriksdóttir - Baddydesign
Illustrations: Bjarney Hinriksdóttir & Istockphotos
Photo image: Alex Eckhart
Proof reader: Will McAuley

The Transformation Journey

A Workbook for Personal Development and Creative Empowerment

First printed edition 2021

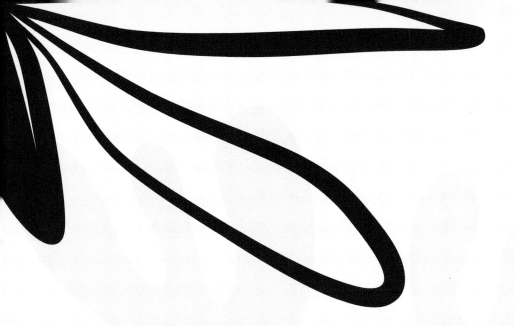

Author's acknowledgement

Just a brief one:

I want to take a moment here and show some gratitude for people who have helped me make this book possible:

First and foremost none of this would have happened without my lifelong best friend and editor, Jodi Marcus. She's a fantastic writer and the most trusted and wonderful friend. We spent more time on the phone on a daily basis during the creation of this book and that in itself was such a great bonus. I hope we have more projects together in the future and continue to make each other laugh until we can't breathe until the end of time!

Without my manager, Myrthe Wieler, and PR manager, Deborah Rossi, I wouldn't be sane. I'm so blessed to have such wonderful, creative and talented women who actually want to work for me. They both go above and beyond the call of duty on a regular basis. Love you guys!

The amazing designer and illustrator, Bjarney Hinriksdóttir (Baddy), is a blessing. Her work really opened up the energy of the book so that it's not just pages of text but brings you into the experience and inspiration.

Am forever grateful for my Dad, William Trano AKA Swami Dadananda. Would I have gone down the path of spirituality and yoga if I hadn't been raised a Vedantist? I'll never know, but his constant dialogue urging me to seek truth has always been a beacon to guide me.

And finally to all the teachers, guides, mentors and holders of wisdom whom I have had the blessing to study with. So much of this book is a testament to the knowledge that these people have passed down and share so graciously with others.

Table of contents

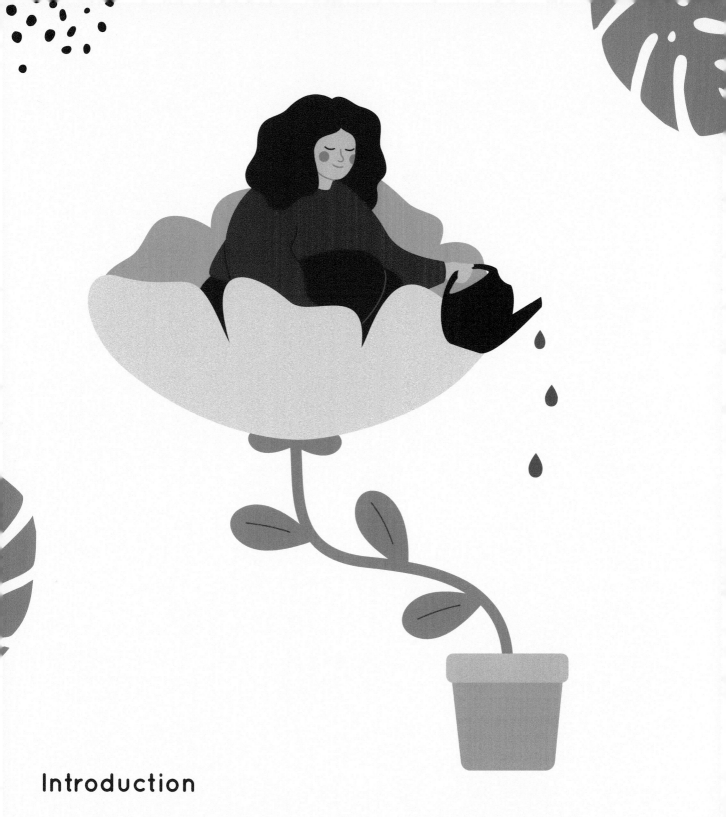

Introduction

You're not alone. Although I know that feeling. That sense that you are totally alone when you're going through a challenging process you don't understand. The end isn't even in sight and everything seems to be conspiring against you. Caught in your head and feeling like an imposter as a lack of self worth creeps into your bones. But let me shed a little light here. Throughout the last 25 years of work bringing yoga, mindful practices and personal development programmes to many places in the world, I've discovered one very profound truth: everyone suffers from a lack of self worth at some point in their lives. Whether long term or short, I've yet to meet anyone who was born with great self awareness and confidence and who is just nailing everything in life. This person doesn't exist!

This is the first and foremost reason I decided to write this book, and I think it's important you understand a little bit about me before we get started on this journey together. I have been through my own process of learning, growing and evolving since I was about 25. I had a difficult relationship with my mother who was controlling and used fear-based parenting skills. It left me feeling suffocated and angry. At that time I had no idea what my belief systems were and I was likely headed for a life of self destruction.

As many good transformations begin, mine started by accident really. Someone had recommended the book You Can Heal Your Life by Louise Hay. Wow, it was the biggest eye opener as I learned that my beliefs and the anger I discovered I was holding onto were causing so much of the pain in my life and my body. I didn't even know that personal development was a thing, but I was totally ripe for it. This was just the beginning, and of course over the years I have been able to redirect my belief systems, let go of the lingering anger, see my self and life through the eyes of curiosity, joy and love. It wasn't easy and I went through a variety of different therapies, techniques, methodologies, theories, and more. But step by step I kept being led, through listening to my inner voice, in the direction of growth, confidence, expansion and healing.

I'm in no way a perfect being, but what I have learned has brought me to the state of clarity and being okay not knowing what is coming next. So, as I discovered how many people were stuck in beliefs of lack or no self worth, I decided to combined the elements and exercises that have helped me the most and continue to help my on my path. I want to share them with everyone in an accessible and sustainable way.

I know change is hard, but when we become tired of our limiting beliefs and self sabotage it's time to begin the journey of transformation. The good news is that everything in this book is practical and applicable. You don't need to be a yogi, although that is my background. The information and inspiration I've gathered here with science and research to back it up comes from some of the most wonderful world renowned teachers and mentors: Brené Brown, Dr Joe Dispenza, Bruce Lipton, Amy Cuddy, Marianne Williamson, Julia Cameron, John Kim and more.

It is my express desire that once you begin this process with me you will unfold and grow into the most fabulous version of yourself.

Julie Martin 2021

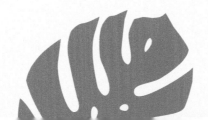

"Make your life a practice of curiosity and you'll never be disappointed."

Julie Martin

I believe in the power of curiosity. Of asking questions. Of going deeper within, rather than seeking answers on the outside. We live in a society that loves to tell us what is right and what is wrong. So we judge ourselves and spend entire lifetimes trying to live up to some expectation of perfection based on someone else's standards.

From my experience this isn't the road to happiness, wholeness, or a life lived from a place of love and authenticity. I suspect you already know this, too, which is why we're together at this juncture.

Let's get all of the "what this workbook isn't" statements out of the way first. This book isn't a "how-to" guide for wellbeing. If it were that simple, we'd all be living the good life after reading a few self-help manuals. Also, this isn't a hippie handbook to "finding your bliss," although it is my sincere hope that the process will help lead you to uncovering greater joy in your life.

This isn't necessarily a book about yoga either, but it does utilise techniques that have sprung out of yoga practices I have used throughout my life. My own curiosity in the relationships between the body, mind, and emotions has led me down many paths - from human movement anatomy to the world of neuroplasticity, from the ancient Vedas to the latest Jeff Foster poems that remind us to be present, patient, and kind to ourselves.

OK, so what are we doing here? Drawing on my years of running yoga teacher trainings, I've realised that if we are truly working with embodiment it has to be about transformation.

I've been on this journey for a while myself. As I continue to travel down these roads again and again, I'm fascinated by and excited to rediscover that transformation is always, well, transformative. With the next breath we move into a new moment with new possibilities, and we can begin once again.

Therefore, this workbook is a map toward initialising that transformation. The journey is yours to explore and it will be different for each individual. As with all good journeys, the road isn't always a straight line. It may be uncomfortable at times and you may feel unsteady, but by using the information, prompts, queries, and tools in this book you will be able to find your way back home - to yourself.

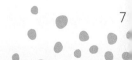

The techniques shared in this workbook have been integral to my own process. I've divided them into three main sections:

Personal Development:

Before we can zoom in on the map and find direction, we'll need to zoom out and look at the whole landscape. This gives us a better understanding of where we are and how we got here. I call the exercises in this section THE 4 PILLARS OF TRANSFORMATION. They will lead you through a progression of self-discovery, involving your own curiosity to ask questions of yourself and your belief systems, and to examine what no longer serves you. Then we can begin to make a map of where we want to be.

Creative Empowerment:

Once we recognise which parts of ourselves we want to nurture and what patterns have held us back, we find a vulnerability. It can be sensitive and fragile, but it will open us up to unveiling our deepest creativity. Our power to create and expand comes from a place beyond judgement, and this section will guide you through that development.

Implementing Growth:

I like to use the word growth as opposed to change. It speaks of a continuous unfolding as opposed to something that is "wrong" with us that needs to be fixed. This section outlines practices to help you continue to evolve and to find new patterns that cultivate a sense of being connected, even when the going gets tough.

As you work through these 3 sections you may find challenge and ease, you may discover things about yourself you hadn't been able to see before. Moments of "ah-ha" or "facepalm". It's all good, it's all process, and it's all a part of life. Each section is designed to support you on your journey, and to give you confidence to continue to believe in yourself.

My goal is that this workbook will bring you to that place of asking: "What is my own personal truth at any moment?", and that by the end of this book you will be able to clearly hear the answers.

Watch video number 1: "Introduction"

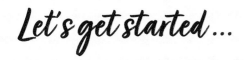
Let's get started ...

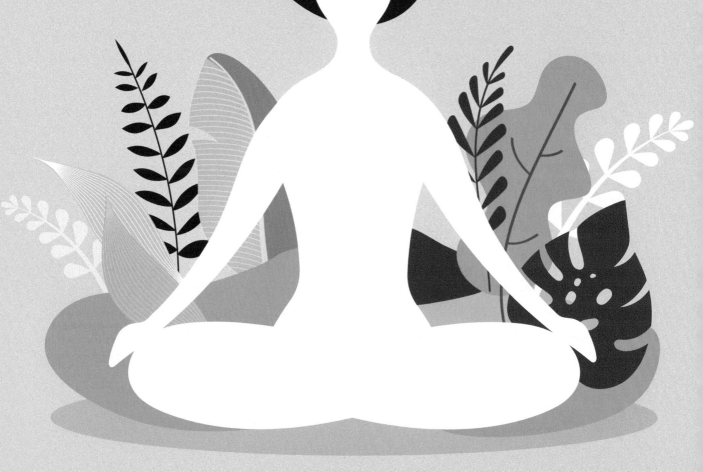

"Knowledge is power,
but knowledge about yourself
is self-empowerment."

Dr. Joe Dispenza

1. Personal development

The Four Pillars of Transformation

The life closet
The First Pillar of Transformation

Start Where You Are is the title of a great book by Pema Chodron. To me, this statement speaks volumes of truth. Let's face it, you can't begin a journey anywhere except where you are right now. It sounds simple, but simple doesn't always mean easy. To help figure out where you are, you're going to take a step back and ask the question: "How did I get here?".

This first exercise will guide you through the process by reorganising what I call your Life Closet. Have you ever noticed how cleaning out a closet is like a trip down memory lane that often leads to some level of clarity? For example, you pull out a shirt or blouse and think "Oh I was wearing this the night so-and-so and I broke up. I learned [BLANK] about myself from that relationship". Or "This is the jacket I wore when I interviewed for my currentjob which now makes me feel [BLANK]".

By unpacking and sorting out the experiences in your Life Closet, you'll examine the parts of your life that have allowed you to arrive at your own personal YOU ARE HERE marker on the map. Think of it as reviewing your present by uncovering, discovering, and discarding that which serves you and that which does not, so you can start your journey from a place of greater insight.

Reorganising your life closet
I know, cleaning out a closet is never fun. It's daunting! It's messy! It's overwhelming! And yet, isn't it always necessary...

So, yes you're going to make a mess. You're going to pull out everything from your Life Closet and spread it all over the place. It's going to seem like a lot of stuff to go through. However, this exercise will allow you to see what may be causing you to feel stuck, frustrated, anxious, and/or confused in order to arrive at a place of understanding "Now I know how I got here".

I've outlined a way to undertake this task by sorting your Life Closet into the containers[1] defined on the next three pages:

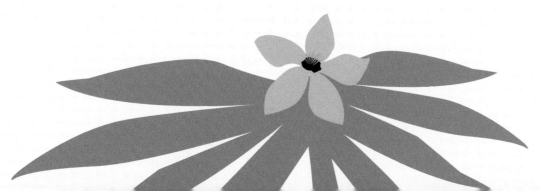

CONTAINER A - Self-Image:

This container will hold your current ideas of who you are. Our self-image is created by our belief systems. All beliefs - whether positive or negative - initially come from somewhere.
As you investigate your self-image remember that it is a collection of influences from many different people and experiences, and that all of these got you to the place where you are now. You might not be aware of how they are operating in your life, and more importantly, they may or may not be speaking your actual truth about yourself.

It can sound a bit new-agey but you are the most important relationship in your life. If there are things you don't like about yourself - for example you recognise a lack of self-worth, suffer from imposter syndrome or have guilt issues - those need to be identified. Also, this container will hold the parts of yourself that you really love or take pride in, and it's necessary to honour these too.

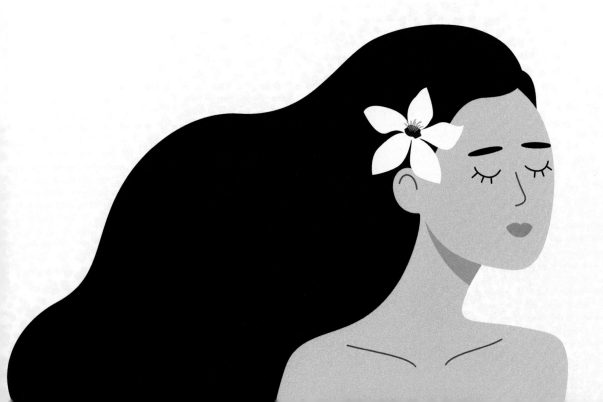

CONTAINER B - Relationships:

Part of being human is having a sense of belonging. It is the opposite of fitting in. Belonging gives you a feeling of safety and connectedness with complete permission to be yourself. We usually encounter a sense of belonging from our family as it holds the most impactful and important relationships in our lives.

As well as family, this container will also hold friendships, romantic relationships, supervisors and/or work colleagues, community members - anyone from a place where a sense of belonging is cultivated.

This container can be challenging as relationships can be highly supportive or they can be the source of some of your biggest obstacles, especially if someone important in your life is linked to one or more limiting belief systems that are projected onto you. This is where you'll detach from the opinions put upon you by others to reveal the authentic you that lies within.

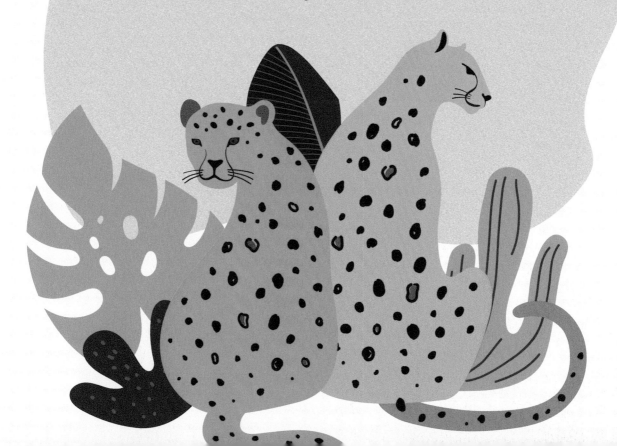

CONTAINER C - Work or Vocation:

"What do you do?", meaning what do you do for a living, is typically the second thing asked upon meeting someone new (right after, "What is your name?"). Your professional life is probably the thing that you primarily use to define yourself, and it most likely takes up the majority of your time, energy, and even much of your mental space. It may influence how you dress, speak, do your hair (or not), etc. In many ways this is where you have the most potential for your voice to be heard out in the world.

But think about it, what you do is just that: what you do. It's not really an indication of who you are as a whole and complete person.

In this container, you'll break down the various aspects of your work life to review what serves you, what might need further examination or even repair, and what is presenting itself as a block.

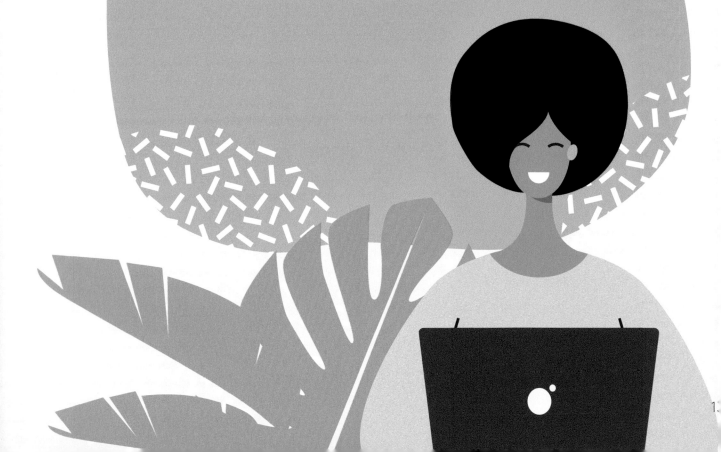

EXERCISE

Now you're going to reorganise your Life Closet container by container. I've outlined 3 different containers above, but you can apply this exercise to any specific area that makes sense to you. You might even just begin with two containers that are super obvious starting points.

There are worksheets on the following pages to make this process easy and clear, with one worksheet per container. Some people/things may show up in more than one container. That's perfectly OK. Remember, this is an examination process and there is no wrong way to do it. My one suggestion is not to overthink it - just let your initial thoughts and gut feelings be your guide.

IMPORTANT:
Fill-in the worksheets by hand and use a pen/pencil.

Complete one container worksheet before moving onto the next.

Go with your gut
(I know I already stated this but it's important enough to be repeated).

Choose one container to work on (Self-Image, Relationships, Work or Vocation). Use the first column labelled "WHAT" to list the things from your Life Closet that belong in that container. [Note: There are no "'should's" here. Just like with a real closet, we're examining what's already there.] Complete this list by filling out the column vertically (top to bottom).

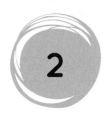

Use the next 3 columns labelled "YAY," "MEH," and "NAY" to assess each person/item listed in column 1. This part is definitely based on how each thing immediately makes you feel when you think about it. Again, complete this step by going from top to bottom. Make a check mark in the appropriate box according to the following system:

YAY - It brings you joy, happiness, pride, etc. These are things that you cherish and fuel you every day. Never underestimate the power of what makes you feel good about yourself. Anything that makes you feel grounded and connected merits a YAY rating.

MEH - You don't have a strong feeling one way or another, or perhaps it is something that used to bring you joy but no longer does. It might need some care and repair, or it might end up in the last column later on. If you feel neutral or undecided about something but it needs some kind of attention, use a MEH rating.

NAY - It makes you feel negative sensations like fear, anger, or resentment. These are things that definitely need to be examined but may no longer serve you. A NAY rating means that this person/thing will be deleted from your LIfe Closet and put into the metaphorical trash.

In the last column labelled "WHY" write a few words or a short sentence about why you rated that person/thing the way that you did. There's no need to go into any depth here, it's just a brief reflection.

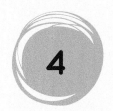
4 Repeat Steps 1 - 3 for the remaining containers.

5 Take some time to sit quietly and see what comes up for you. If your inner voice conflicts with what you initially put on the page, review the rating you gave it and the reasons why, and make any changes that you feel reveal a deeper truth.

6 Leave this exercise for a few days and see if you notice things pop into your head in relation to what you have written down.

See the following page for a sample of this exercise.

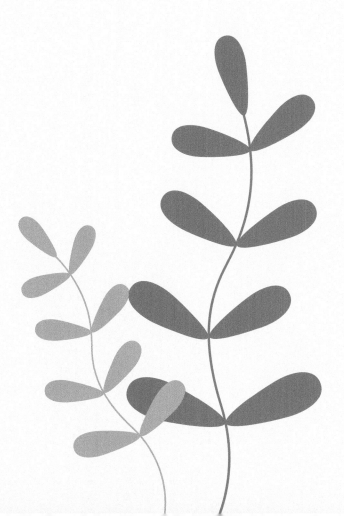

SELF-IMAGE CONTAINER

WHAT	YAY	MEH	NAY	WHY
YOGA PRACTITIONER		X		I FEEL LIKE AN IMPOSTER SOMETIMES IN MY LOCAL YOGA CLASS, BUT I LOVE HOW THE PRACTICE MAKES ME FEEL.
BODY IMAGE		X		I LIKE HOW MY BODY MOVES AND FEELS BUT WORRY ABOUT GETTING OLDER AND NOT FEELING AS MUCH ENERGY AS I USED TO.
MOTHER	X			I LOVE BEING A MOM AND MY KIDS GIVE ME A GREAT SENSE OF PRIDE.
SELF CRITICISM			X	MY SELF TALK IS OFTEN NEGATIVE AND MAKES ME PROCRASTINATE DOING THINGS I THINK I'D REALLY ENJOY

NOTE: If this exercise seems too vulnerable, it may be helpful to imagine that your best friend is answering these questions for you. We can often be overly self-critical (which may be something to examine in your Self-Image container), but when we see ourselves through the lens of someone who knows us well and unconditionally has our back, we notice our assets and beauty better than when left to our own self-judgement.

CONTAINER A - Self Image

WHAT	YAY	MEH	NAY	WHY

CONTAINER B - Relationships

WHAT	YAY	MEH	NAY	WHY

CONTAINER C - Work or Vocation

WHAT	YAY	MEH	NAY	WHY

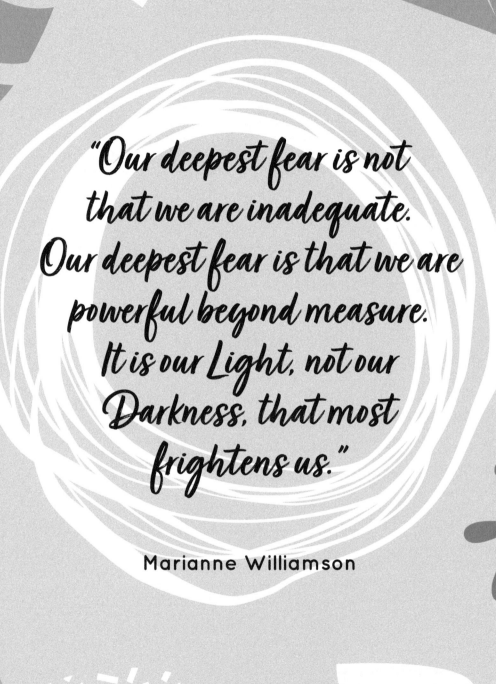

"Our deepest fear is not that we are inadequate. Our deepest fear is that we are powerful beyond measure. It is our Light, not our Darkness, that most frightens us."

Marianne Williamson

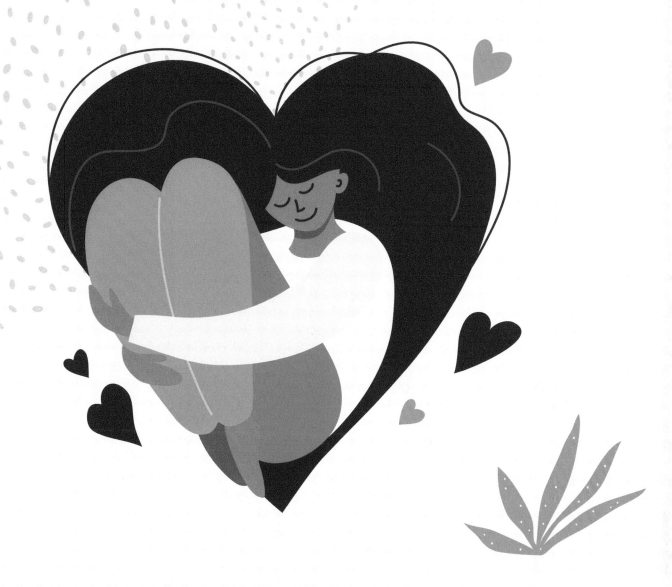

The gratitude journal of manifestation

The Second Pillar of Transformation

You might notice how easy it is to talk about what you don't want. To make lists of things in your head that you are trying to stop doing or want to get rid of. This is why we did the Life Closet exercise. But we can't begin the transformation process until we know what it is that we truly do want.

This brings us to an examination of gratitude. It seems like I can't be on social media for more than five minutes without coming across a post about it. I think this is great, but I often wonder if these posts might just be feigning an "attitude of gratitude," as opposed to being a tool for deeply connecting us with what we are grateful for. I'm talking about the ability to cherish what we have, what we've been through, and even what is uncertain or scary.

Moreover, if we want to create some growth in our lives we have to approach our intentions with gratitude before they even happen. Sounds a bit odd maybe? But stick with me as we undertake the Second Pillar of Transformation: the Gratitude Journal.

I've used this exercise in all of my teacher trainings, and it is pretty amazing how much it helps to stimulate transformation. This isn't your average gratitude journal where you take time every day to write about what you're thankful for. Although that is a very useful exercise and part of this practice, this Gratitude Journal is about moving into the future with an energy of gratitude for what is coming next.

The Universe connects to our energy in relation to what we're focused on. Therefore, if we're focused on what we don't want, it generates more of the same. This is why we can finish one relationship or job thinking we're done with "that business/mistake", only to find ourselves in a similar situation once again. Conversely, the Universe responds to meaningful and positive petitions as well. Ever have a "synchronicity" happen when you least expected it? The important question is: "What do we really want?".

Before embarking on this exercise, it's necessary to identify a higher power to whom you are expressing your gratitude. It can be God, the gods, the goddesses, the Universe, the Divine Creator or any other name that works for you. It just needs to feel comfortable and authentic to you and your connection.

> *Practising gratitude is how we acknowledge that there's enough and that we're enough."*
>
> **Brené Brown**

EXERCISE

Start with a blank journal book. Open to the second page so that there is a blank sheet on the left side and a blank sheet on the right.

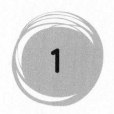

THE LEFT SIDE - Gratitude for what you do have

On the left side of the page write 5 things that you are grateful for that are in your life right now. It can be big things (having a life partner) and small things (that delicious cookie you just ate). It can be good things that happen to you and bad things that turned out to be good things later. You can write the same thing every day, come up with completely different things, or use a combination of repeated and new statements. Again, this is your Gratitude Journal and there are no wrong answers.

Notice how you feel. Maybe you even find yourself smiling while you write. Pause after writing each sentence and really feel that gratitude in your body.

THE RIGHT SIDE - What are you manifesting

As you may have guessed, the right side of the page will be used to write 5 things that you want to have in your life. However, manifesting isn't about having positive thoughts and setting intentions. It's not about concrete details, either. It's much deeper than that. It's about getting to the true core of what you really want. You may think that you want something but when you start to get too specific you might realise that you actually missed the mark, and that you accidentally manifested something very unwanted.

Let me give you a slightly gruesome but very clear example:

Say you want to lose 3 kilos. You may start writing "I'm so deeply grateful to the Universe that my body is 3 kilos lighter and I didn't have to go on a crazy diet". Now take a look at your forearm. How much do you think it weighs? Probably about 3 kilos. If you got into an accident and damaged your forearm so badly it had to be removed you'd lose 3 kilos.

I use this example because many women feel dissatisfied with their bodies, and they often look at weight as the main thing they are unhappy about. But looking at the manifestation statement above and at possible outcomes we see that it isn't about losing 3 kilos. This is where the clarity comes in (as opposed to specific details). It's not the weight. What we want to manifest is; I feel so deeply grateful to the Universe that I love my body exactly the way it is - healthy, strong, mobile, and filled with youthful energy. This is what we're really and truly looking for, right?

As you begin to write the 5 things you are manifesting, understand that it might take a few days or even a week to refine the clarity. It's important to keep in mind the following:

- **The Universe gets confused by negative statements**
  For example: "I'm so deeply grateful to the Universe that I no longer feel bad about my job and don't have to interact with my co-workers".

- **Avoid predicting the outcome**
  Continuing with the example above: "...and that I get a promotion by the end of the month". When we predict the outcome we close off possibilities. Often the outcome arrives in a very unexpected way. If it was predictable you would have already done it, had it, been there.

Based on the example above, here's a reframe: "I'm so deeply grateful to the Universe that I have a job that's fulfilling and utilises my talents well, where I work with kind and creative colleagues, and I earn more money than I dreamed of".

For this side, it will be helpful to look at the "MEH" and "NAY" columns from your Life Closet. These are areas where you might want to find growth or re-define what better supports the authentic you. You may have discovered a self-belief that no longer serves you and this is where you can write the opposite belief, i.e. changing "lack" into "abundance."

Let's take another example; suppose that you are unhappy in your relationship with your partner. This would be an example of what to write on the right side: "I'm so deeply grateful to the Universe that I'm in a romantic relationship with someone who sees me as a whole and amazing person, encourages me and also challenges me in positive ways, and with whom we can grow together emotionally and spiritually".

What this statement does is eliminate names or projection onto your current partner. What tends to happen is that you may find your current partner beginning to change his/her behaviour to match what you are manifesting.

Alternatively, you may find your partner becoming more agitated and indifferent and the relationship gets worse. This is usually a sign from the Universe that you're with the wrong person for what you want in your life. You may split up, but then you are open to receiving a new partner who does offer what you really want in a relationship. Remember, we can't change other people but we can be clear about what we really want to manifest and see what the Universe provides.

NOTE: All statements are written in the present moment. Things you are manifesting are written as if you already have them. No different in language than writing on the left side. Avoid using the term "I want...." as the minute you state you "want" something you've told the Universe that you don't have it. Since the only moment we have is right now, our energy will respond to our statements as if we already have what we are seeking. When that energy is in motion the Universe provides. It might not happen the way you think it should, so be prepared for surprises, but it will come your way.

When completing either side, it's perfectly OK to review what you have written on previous days. In fact, I encourage it. You'll find the left side to be easier to do. Remember the right side will take some time to refine. Ask yourself after each statement: "Is this true? Is this really what I want to manifest?". Once you clarify your statements you'll find your truth and recognise it. Then repeat the statement the same way every day until it's delivered by the Universe. Once that happens you can write it on the left side of your journal. What's important is that you remain open to the possibilities.

IMPORTANT:
Write this journal by hand and use a pen/pencil.

Write in full sentences, as opposed to just listing things, and be descriptive. For example:
"I'm so grateful to the Universe for my beautiful community of friends and family who give me support when I need it and have my back unconditionally".

Start with 5 statements on the left and 5 statements on the right. It's OK if you want to do more, just be sure there is an equal number on each side. I suggest a maximum of 10 statements per side.

Do this exercise daily and at the same time of day, if possible. For example, set aside 20 minutes first thing in the morning, or use this as a closing exercise before going to sleep.

The following are just a few examples to give a clearer picture. If one or more resonates with you use it as a template and then create a more personal description. Remember not to use specific names or places, jobs, etc. as our greatest good might lie elsewhere.

Watch video number 2: "Gratitude Journal"

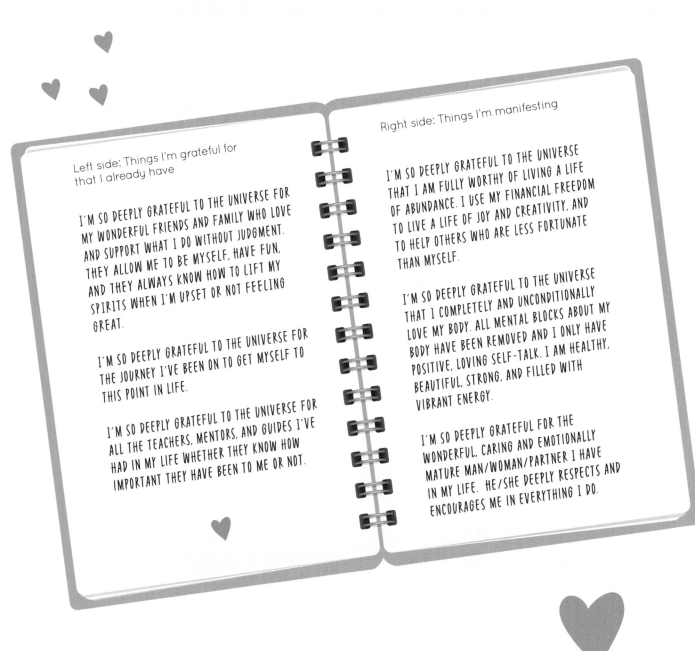

Left side: Things I'm grateful for that I already have

I'M SO DEEPLY GRATEFUL TO THE UNIVERSE FOR MY WONDERFUL FRIENDS AND FAMILY WHO LOVE AND SUPPORT WHAT I DO WITHOUT JUDGMENT. THEY ALLOW ME TO BE MYSELF, HAVE FUN, AND THEY ALWAYS KNOW HOW TO LIFT MY SPIRITS WHEN I'M UPSET OR NOT FEELING GREAT.

I'M SO DEEPLY GRATEFUL TO THE UNIVERSE FOR THE JOURNEY I'VE BEEN ON TO GET MYSELF TO THIS POINT IN LIFE.

I'M SO DEEPLY GRATEFUL TO THE UNIVERSE FOR ALL THE TEACHERS, MENTORS, AND GUIDES I'VE HAD IN MY LIFE WHETHER THEY KNOW HOW IMPORTANT THEY HAVE BEEN TO ME OR NOT.

Right side: Things I'm manifesting

I'M SO DEEPLY GRATEFUL TO THE UNIVERSE THAT I AM FULLY WORTHY OF LIVING A LIFE OF ABUNDANCE. I USE MY FINANCIAL FREEDOM TO LIVE A LIFE OF JOY AND CREATIVITY, AND TO HELP OTHERS WHO ARE LESS FORTUNATE THAN MYSELF.

I'M SO DEEPLY GRATEFUL TO THE UNIVERSE THAT I COMPLETELY AND UNCONDITIONALLY LOVE MY BODY. ALL MENTAL BLOCKS ABOUT MY BODY HAVE BEEN REMOVED AND I ONLY HAVE POSITIVE, LOVING SELF-TALK. I AM HEALTHY, BEAUTIFUL, STRONG, AND FILLED WITH VIBRANT ENERGY.

I'M SO DEEPLY GRATEFUL FOR THE WONDERFUL, CARING AND EMOTIONALLY MATURE MAN/WOMAN/PARTNER I HAVE IN MY LIFE. HE/SHE DEEPLY RESPECTS AND ENCOURAGES ME IN EVERYTHING I DO.

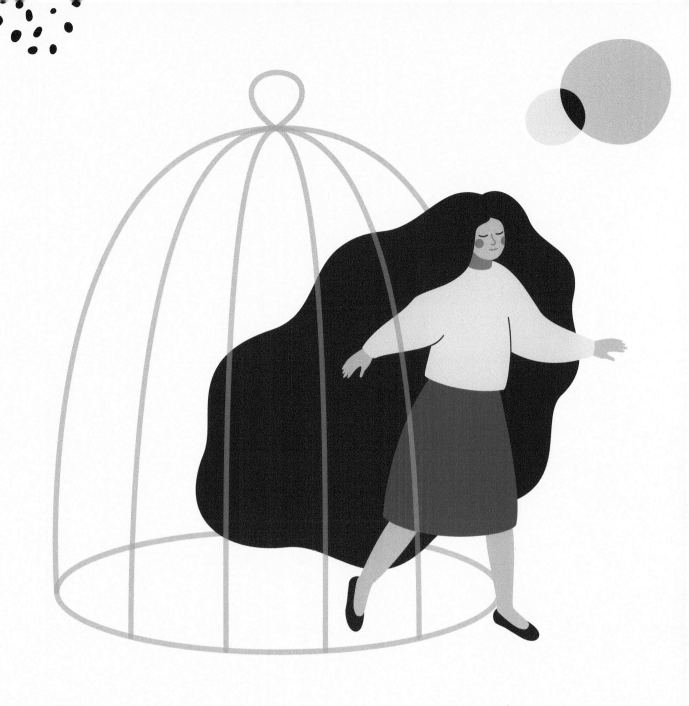

Redirecting belief systems
The Third Pillar of Transformation

As you move through the first two Pillars, you'll uncover which belief systems hold you back the most. They may have been with you a lifetime or they may have crept up more recently due to circumstances. Perhaps you've been doing this kind of work for a while and you wonder why it feels like it would be easier to move a brick wall rather than change an old negative belief system. You're not alone and you're not at fault. We're actually wired in our brains to keep our thought/sensation patterns on a continuous loop, regardless of whether they are helpful or harmful. This is why the same limiting beliefs keep filtering into our thoughts - and by extension into our bodies - thus influencing our life outcomes.

Here's a bit of science to further explain how this works:

Information based on emotion (fear, anxiety, joy, relaxation, etc.) is processed in the brain's limbic system. When we have an experience that creates a strong emotional sensation, like anger or elation, the limbic system records our emotional response. As with all parts of the body, the limbic system prefers to operate with efficiency. Therefore, when we repeatedly encounter a similar experience, the limbic system will bypass the conscious thought process and automatically create the remembered sensations in the body.

What this means is that each time we are in a similarly stressful situation or even have a negative recurring thought about something, the limbic system goes into auto-mode and releases the same level of stress hormone (cortisol) into our bodies. The limbic system keeps this repeated loop on auto-dial.

For example, if you grew up in a family that consistently reminded you that "money doesn't grow on trees," every time you're faced with a financial situation your limbic system will trigger the same sensation of how that lack feels in the body, typically causing fear and/or anxiety. This automatically releases a preset level of cortisol into the system. So your cells are remembering, reinforcing, and reliving that sensation of lack as it relates to money.

If we could change our limbic system just by thinking better thoughts we'd all be healthy, happy, in love, and living in abundance. However, since it's our limbic system's job to create an emotional loop (as opposed to cognitive thought), we have to change our emotion first in order to arrive at a different response.

Something else to consider: when we try to force our thoughts and responses to change by utilising fear, shame, anxiety, etc., we just end up laying down more pathways of fear, shame or anxiety. That's because using force causes the nervous system to say there's something wrong with the organism (us). Therefore, we're putting more negative energy into a negative response, and producing a repeated negative outcome. This is why we can't hate our bodies into thinness. Or complain about a lack of money to make ourselves rich. Or focus on our partner's shortcomings to create a healthy relationship.

For all of these reasons, the Third Pillar is about *redirection*. We want to utilise our awareness (mind) and our energy (body) for transformation. So how do we redirect our body's auto-response? We literally have to rewire our brain (See Resources: Dr. Joe Dispenza).

Don't worry, you don't need to be a scientist to figure this out. It's not as complicated as it might sound. The brain doesn't know the difference between something we're just remembering and something that's happening right now. This is why mentally reliving a joyous occasion or an argument, even if it happened years ago, will trigger the same emotions and sensations in the body that you felt on that day. The key is to change the emotion to our desired outcome *before* we even experience it. The exercises at the end of this chapter will help to redirect your focus, guide you into cultivating emotions that match the sensations of love, abundance, productivity, happiness, etc., and move you away from replaying and analysing the "why me" thoughts that reiterate the negative response.

Here's a real-life example of how this works:

I have a friend who's belief system told her that she had to be perfect all of the time - from her career, to a yoga pose, to cleaning the toilet, and everything in between. Her identity was totally wrapped up in this unhealthy belief system. Even when she understood that her perfectionism was causing tremendous unhappiness, she was terrified to let up on herself. By desperately clinging to what was known (*I have to be perfect in everything I do or I don't know how to exist*) she ended up burnt out at the height of her career, hurting herself in yoga, and neglecting to clean her home because it took way too long.

In her effort to be perfect at everything, she became trapped in an emotional and physical loop that prevented her from ever feeling relaxed, joy, or true connection with herself or with others.

She now calls herself a "recovering perfectionist," but what she's really doing is detoxing from the deeply ingrained belief that she has to be perfect in order to feel safe, and from the high levels of cortisol that belief system produced in her body over so many years. She's redirecting the thought and the sensation of "I have to be perfect all of the time" to "I'm good enough just as I am". Today, she has left her job to pursue her creative endeavours, does yoga as an embodied practice, and is more present to her loved ones.

When we rewire our brains we redirect ourselves in three ways:

1. Our minds become liberated from the attachment to our limiting belief systems as:
2. Our bodies detox from the addiction to being on high levels of cortisol activated by those belief systems, and;
3. We strengthen our physical and mental wellbeing since high levels of cortisol suppress our immune system.

"We cannot create a new future holding on to the emotions of the past"

Dr. Joe Dispenza

Let's examine some categories of belief systems in order to understand where they came from, how they've shaped our current identity, and why some of them will be more challenging to shift.

Categories of Belief Systems

Inherited beliefs

These are beliefs instilled in us from our outside worlds: culture, society, family, etc. Because their roots are long, these beliefs are more challenging to overcome. The critical thing to understand is that they aren't yours to begin with. You need to see them as a separate entity outside of yourself. Like an old fur coat inherited from your great-grandma. It might have been a lovely thing for her, but do you really need it? Or even want it?

A perfect example of this is the aforementioned feeling of lack as it relates to money. If your parents, grandparents, and previous generations had fears and/or anxiety about money, it's highly likely that you grew up with an inherited mindset of lack. You may have heard your parents' conversations about money being tight, there's never enough, and it's always hard-earned. You may have repeated similar sentences to your children or friends, thinking and feeling that this stress around finances is normal. Even if you have a really lucrative job you can still operate from the emotions of scarcity because they are embedded in your limbic system.

Inherited Belief
I'll never have a lot of money.

Redirected Belief
I am worthy of abundance.

Childhood Inflicted

Whether they're delivered by a parent, a school teacher, a sibling, or friends, ideas about our capabilities are usually formulated in the first 7 years of our lives. Perhaps an incident at school or with your siblings had such a strong emotional charge that became set in stone. Encounters with a bully or harsh words from a misguided teacher can formulate a belief system that sticks with us our entire lives - until we notice it and challenge it.

In my own experience, I was often made to feel like I wasn't very smart. My parents told me that as long as I earned a "C" in a class that was fine, and my teachers never pushed me either. By the time I was a teenager my self-belief was *"I'm not smart"*. However, as a young adult, after high school and beyond, I learned that I loved to read, I'm great at problem-solving, I can fully understand and explain complex ideas, and I can clearly see the big picture about things. Once I noticed my abilities, I could experience the sensation of being smart as if someone told me they were impressed with my intelligence, and I released those childhood inflicted beliefs. From there, I was able to create a thriving business (having never been to business school), confidently speak in public (without any formal training), and manage up to 16 staff (without taking any management courses).

Childhood Belief
I'm told I'm not talented enough to become a (writer, dancer, singer, yoga teacher, etc.).

Redirected Belief
I am my own distinct set of experiences, abilities, and skills that makes me uniquely talented to be a (writer, dancer, singer, yoga teacher, etc.).

Adult Traumatic Incident
These are incidents that happen later in life but still trigger a belief system in the body. They are often linked to an unexpected and unpleasant life-changing event, like losing a job, a close family member, or getting divorced.

For example, perhaps you were in a wonderful relationship that seemed like it was for the long term, until you discovered that your husband/wife/ partner was cheating on you. And maybe that led to an ugly and toxic divorce. This is a traumatic incident that can shatter your self-confidence and make it difficult to trust in potential new partners. If you hold onto the anger, resentment, and even the cruel words of your ex long after the relationship has ended, this can become a deeply embedded belief system. You are very likely to enter into any new romantic relationship with those same emotions.

Adult Traumatic Belief
I can't trust my choices or my new partner because the last one cheated on me.

Redirected Belief
I am worthy of a being in a loving and committed relationship.

"*Wherever your awareness goes is where your energy flows.*"

Dr. Joe Dispenza

Now it's time to override the limbic system by putting some higher vibrations into our practice. Remember, this isn't necessarily going to be easy because some of these beliefs may have been in your body since before cognitive memory. But now that you understand a bit of the science behind why it's been difficult to change, you can redirect your efforts. The following 3 exercises lay the foundation for this process.

EXERCISES

Re-examine Your Gratitude Journal
Review the things you're working on manifesting that are included on the right side of your Gratitude Journal. Re-read each statement separately and notice if there are any sensations, thoughts, or memories that arise. If you have a negative feeling, ask yourself if there is a belief system in the background that may be preventing you from having already achieved that outcome. Remind yourself that the negative belief system is no longer yours and you don't need to own it. Then rephrase what it is you want to manifest in order to redirect the belief system.

Example: Perhaps you've been writing about owning your dream home. Quietly ask yourself: "Do I feel worthy of this?" or "Am I deserving?" If the underlying answer that arises is No, I'll never afford it then it's necessary to talk to the limbic system. Before you can manifest your dream home you need to feel that you are worthy of abundance. Write on the right side of your journal; "I'm so deeply grateful to the Universe that I am worthy of abundance and deserve everything I desire", and then pause to generate a feeling of abundance by imagining what it would feel like if you knew you could have everything you dreamed of. Imagine you have full access to the Universal Trust Fund.

The Universal Trust Fund
There is a great abundance that exists in the world. There is in fact enough money, food, space, etc. for everyone on this planet. It's the natural order of balance. But we hear about lack more than anything so that's what we believe. In order to cultivate the energy of abundance ask yourself: "What would it feel if I had access to an unlimited trust fund that I could use anytime I like?". How would you feel, behave, go about your day? This is the energy you want to project.

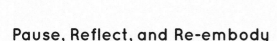

Pause, Reflect, and Re-embody

As you go through your day take notice when you react to something and/or you hear yourself using language that no longer aligns with who you want to be. Understand that this is triggered by your old belief system. Pause, ground yourself, and deepen your breath. Reflect by telling yourself: That was the old belief. Re-embody by asking yourself: *How would I feel and behave right now if I believed X* (insert new belief system).

Example: If you believed that you were living in abundance, you would change your phrasing from "I can't afford that" to "That is not going to fulfill me right now". Rephrasing our thoughts and language around the concept that has been holding us back opens the doorway to a different feeling. Notice that it's not about going ahead and buying something if you're feeling lack (although I have a little story about that below and if the item would indeed fulfill you then it might be wise to go ahead and commit to buying it). It's about rewiring the circuit in the brain that says "I can't afford it" and the sensation that arises with that thought.

My little story: Many years ago when I was first introduced to this understanding via Louise Hay's book *You Can Heal Your Life* I was excited but also hesitant. I wanted to be "all in" but I wasn't sure nor did I have the scientific explanation yet about how our brains work. One day, I went to the ATM to discover that I only had about £100 in my account to last the rest of the month (it was around the 15th). I could feel the sensation of fear creep in around not having enough money. Then I had my *Pause and Redirect* moment. I thought to myself, "OK how can I change this?"

I'm definitely a "go big or go home" kind of person, so instead of just rephrasing my thought, I jumped on a bus to the shopping area of town (Brighton, UK) and headed straight to Karen Millen (a rather posh clothing store that specialises in tailoring, coats, jackets, etc.). I had always walked past the store window afraid to actually go in let alone even try on something. But on that day, I opened the door and immediately caught sight of a gorgeous, bright red, faux fur coat with a leopard-print lining. It was stunning! It was audacious! It was not even remotely about function or a sensible purchase! And it was £500! I tried it on, loved how I felt in it, and decided right then and there, "This is mine!" I took out my credit card and wore that coat on the bus home feeling like a queen. I did not feel any guilt, shame, or anxiety after buying that coat. I felt great. I felt like I deserved it. And I slept well that night.

In the morning I got a call from a man who had been given my number by another yoga teacher. He was looking for someone to teach for an hour each morning on a management training course to help the participants get into their bodies and out of their heads. It was for 5 days, an hour each morning. The pay? £100 per hour. I hung up the phone, laughed myself silly, looked up at the sky out the window, and shouted, "OK, I get it!"

"Everytime you overcome the voices that tell you to make decisions that are not ultimately loving to you, you are applying your conscious will over your body & you conquer an aspect of yourself."

- Dr. Joe Dispenza

Redirection Meditation

Meditation is one of the best ways to really connect to the feelings and emotions created in our bodies by our belief systems. This can be used as an add-on to whatever current meditation practice you already have. There are no rules and regulations because this is about your own experience.

If you don't already have a meditation practice, start by finding a comfortable seat and relax. Notice what's connecting you to the ground (you can sit on a chair or directly on the floor). Let your awareness travel up the body. Notice your spine, your shoulders, arms, hands, head. Be aware of how it feels to be sitting. Relax the throat by swallowing. Check with your eyebrows and forehead to make sure there is no tension. Then just observe your breath. Notice the breath as it is. Don't try to change it, but if it does start to become slower and deeper then let it. You can do this for 2-3 minutes as an opener to the meditation below. You can continue to read the instructions below or go straight to the guided meditation in the video.

Watch video number 3: "Meditation-Redirecting Beliefs"

- Think about the belief you'd like to transform and notice the sensations that arise in your body when you initially think about the old belief system.

- Recognise the old belief as just that: a belief, a thought, something that can change.

- Next, think about the new belief system you'd like to "install." How does this feel in your body?

- Your limbic system will probably pipe up and argue or try to distract you with other thoughts. Don't worry, that's normal. Notice it and return to the new belief system.

- Envision yourself doing amazing things within the new belief system. How would you feel? How would you behave? Notice the emotion that arises. Cultivate an elevated positive emotion and fill your body with this new sensation.

- See how long you can sit there in that positive sensation. Embrace it with your being. Feel it beyond your skin.

- Repeat the new belief to yourself over and over again while feeling the new emotion.

Example:

Suppose you're cultivating a new belief system around self-worth. Get into your meditation, think about your new belief system, and say to yourself, "I'm worthy of [BLANK]". If the limbic system runs its old loop of thoughts and sensations (and it will), simply notice them, and return to thinking, "I am worthy". Cultivate what that feels like in your body. If it's challenging to create a positive sensation, think of someone or something that fills you with complete joy. Understand that your joy comes from a place of love that is powerful and abundant, and that you deserve to feel it unconditionally. Embrace this sensation with your entire being. You might even end up smiling in your mediation because this is the limbic system taking note. Repeat to yourself, "I am worthy" again and again while you're feeling that new emotion.

Try to sustain this new sensation for as long as you can. It may be for only a few minutes in the beginning, and that's great. Try to work up to 10-15 minutes. This is how you stamp the sensation and the belief onto your cells so that when you get up from your meditation you're likely to feel empowered, amazing, and in love with life. During the day, whenever you feel yourself returning to your old beliefs remind yourself of what you experienced in your meditation, recapture it, and congratulate yourself for it.

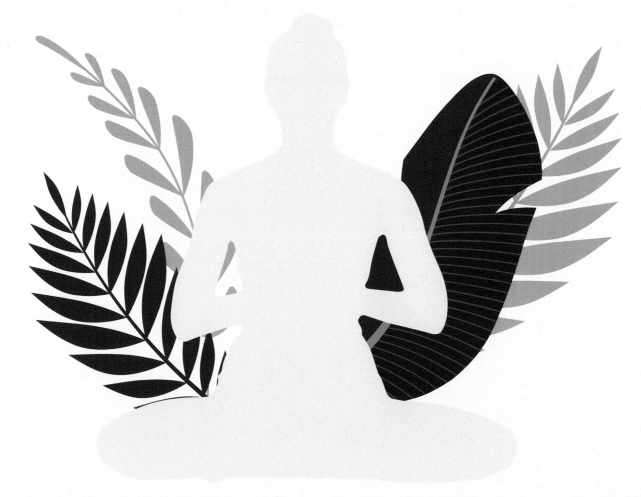

"There's nothing more powerful than a woman who knows how to contain her power and not let it leak, standing firmly within it in mystery and 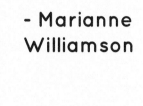 silence."

- Marianne Williamson

Yourself as a superhero
The Fourth Pillar of Transformation

This Pillar is all about creating the *Power You* as a tool to tap into when you're working on changing those old beliefs and limitations. Who do you want to be when you wake up in the morning? Which superpowers would you have? It can be anything from always being on time to running a marathon. These superpowers should dovetail with the new belief system you're cultivating. If it's abundance, then what do you imagine a person living in abundance does in their daily life? Or if it's finding love and deeply connecting to a partner, what powers do you have as the super version of yourself in a relationship?

Dream big or small, but putting together a vision of yourself as a Superhero gives you direction and potential for thriving. Our Superheroes are all about embodying the elevated emotions we're creating. When we experience joy, gratitude, confidence, and self-empowerment we are feeling those higher vibrations, and this is the opportunity to talk to the body at a cellular level. We affirm the new belief systems/emotions as if we already have them. We are living them right now; we believe in ourselves right now. Your Superhero knows you can't fail, you can only find new ways to learn and to grow.

The key question in this section is: "What would I do and how would I behave if I was ALREADY the person I really want to be?" We need to shift the paradigm to the present moment. And this is why creating your own Superhero is a vital tool. It may feel like a game at first, but you'll discover that once you get the hang of it you can tap into your Superhero whenever you need to. Over time you realise you're already there. You become your Superhero.

Building Your Superhero Toolkit

If you're feeling a lack of self-worth or confidence, or your negative self-talk around money issues arising, or your imposter syndrome's chattering on and you're having a hard time creating your new emotional state, the exercises below are about empowering yourself and embodying your Superhero. Have fun with this section. When you're enjoying yourself in the process then you're already working from a higher vibration. If anything brings laughter into the mix, that's even better. Invite a friend to join you. Your shared elevated emotions will be infectious.

Power Playlist

Pick 4 or 5 songs that really uplift you and get you grooving. The ones that make you want to dance, sing at the top of your lungs, jump on your bed. The lyrics express a deep "YES!" from within and make you want to punch the air, be a rockstar, or imagine yourself flying high.

Listen to your Power Playlist on the way to meetings or prior to teaching a class, before going on a date, or any time you feel doubt trickling into your body. When I find myself scrolling on social media too long or procrastinating about completing some task, I put on my Power Playlist and go for a walk which often turns into dancing, skipping, and singing to the animals as I pass by (I live where there are a lot of cows and horses). My energy soars and I have moments of feeling absolutely invincible. Then I take a moment to create a memory of these feelings, so that it becomes a mental/visceral photograph I can revisit.

If you love dancing like no one is watching, then this practice can be enormously powerful for you. Joyous movement will automatically lower cortisol levels while releasing dopamine, oxytocin, serotonin, and endorphins (D.O.S.E.) that have lasting effects even hours after you've finished dancing.

"There are so many studies done around dance and happiness and the science of dance as a healing modality. It's the most healing modality that exists on the planet. When you dance, it releases your DOSE."

Radha Agrawal

Power Posing and Power Mantra

Power Posing comes from Amy Cuddy's work (See Resources). In brief, Power Posing is about the effect our physical stance has on our mood and emotions. If our posture has been hunched over a computer all day with our shoulders dropping forward, we often feel tired, closed off, and heavy. When we place our bodies into a shape that represents confidence, for example standing upright with hands on our hips, we automatically begin to *feel* spacious and confident. Think of postures or actions that athletes naturally do when they score a goal or cross a finish line. They're big, they're bold, and they're universal. When we make these same poses, our emotions follow the expression of the body.

To find your own Power Poses think of words or phrases to describe how you want to feel. Then ask your body what those words would look like if they were shapes. Play around with this a few times. Have your Power Playlist on to make it even easier.

Move through your Power Pose shapes over and over again, narrowing them down to 2 or 3. Repeat them a few times. The body and the mind start to link up as you repeat. Your words or phrases become Power Mantras like *"I am amazing!"*, *"I can do this!"* or *"I am worthy!"*. Combine these with your Power Playlist and a good crazy ass dance around the house, and you'll cultivate fully embodied and elevated emotions.

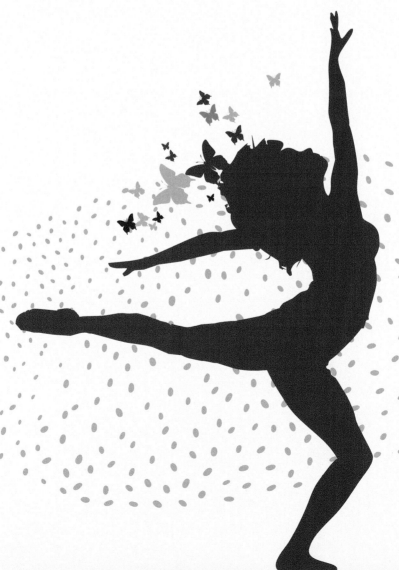

Take a moment to notice how your body feels in these shapes. Make a visceral photograph. Now you'll have the capability to feel this way whenever you want to. Do your Power Poses and Power Mantra for 2-3 minutes just before a tough conversation with someone who triggers your old belief systems, while getting ready for a job interview, a date, or a big presentation, or when you're about to make a large purchase. If you're somewhere where you can't comfortably move into your Power Poses, then just stand quietly in a private space (like a restroom) and visualise yourself going through them. Mentally recall your Power Mantra. Smile to yourself and see how you feel now.

Power Costume
We all have an outfit, dress, jeans, top, or even a piece of jewelry or an accessory that just makes us feel really good when we wear it. Maybe it's because the colour makes your eyes pop, you feel sexy and/or slimmer in it, or you like the way it makes your bum look. If you don't currently have a favourite article of clothing or an outfit that gives you that feeling, invest in something (Remember my little story about that flaming red faux fur coat? Oh yes!). It doesn't have to be expensive, it just needs to be something that you feel great wearing.

Creating your Power Costume and wearing it can do wonders to elevate your mood. You might even have two Power Costumes (casual and dressy). Wear them often, especially if you're feeling down and/or lack energy. We often put on drabby clothes when we're having a crappy day, but wearing something we feel good in can bring that boost of confidence that's needed. And remember, if someone compliments you just say thank you. No excuses, no saying, "This old thing?" or "I look a mess". It's too common in society to be told not to stand out or to show that you feel good about yourself. This is what gave us our negative beliefs in the first place. Own your beauty and your individuality. And make it a practice to compliment others when you notice something unique about them - it will also make you feel good too.

If you want to have more fun with this and love feeling flamboyant, you may even decide to make a full on Superhero Costume! Go all out and get a crown, glitter, those thigh high boots that you can't even walk in. Maybe you just wear this around your house, or you throw a party and invite all of your friends to create their own Superhero Costumes, and see what happens. Encourage everyone to arrive as the best version of themselves.

Extra advice: If part of your Power Costume is a simple top or jeans that's easy to buy, get one or two extra, maybe in different colours. Steve Jobs was famous for wearing the same thing everyday. He worked with fashion designer Issey Miyake to create a standard look that he felt comfortable and empowered in, ordered dozens of the same top (black mock turtleneck) and jeans, so that he never had to think about what he was going to wear but knew that he would feel confident each day.

And just one more note of advice, be careful that your Power Costume speaks to your authenticity as opposed to being a layer of armour to preserve a negative belief in disguise (literally!). Ask yourself: "Do I feel free, uplifted and empowered in this?". I'll refer back to my "recovering perfectionist" friend who used to wear buttoned-up, fitted clothes, and high heels even as her casual wear to project a certain image based on her negative belief, and now goes around in loose t-shirts, flowing trousers, and flat shoes to express her real and authentic self.

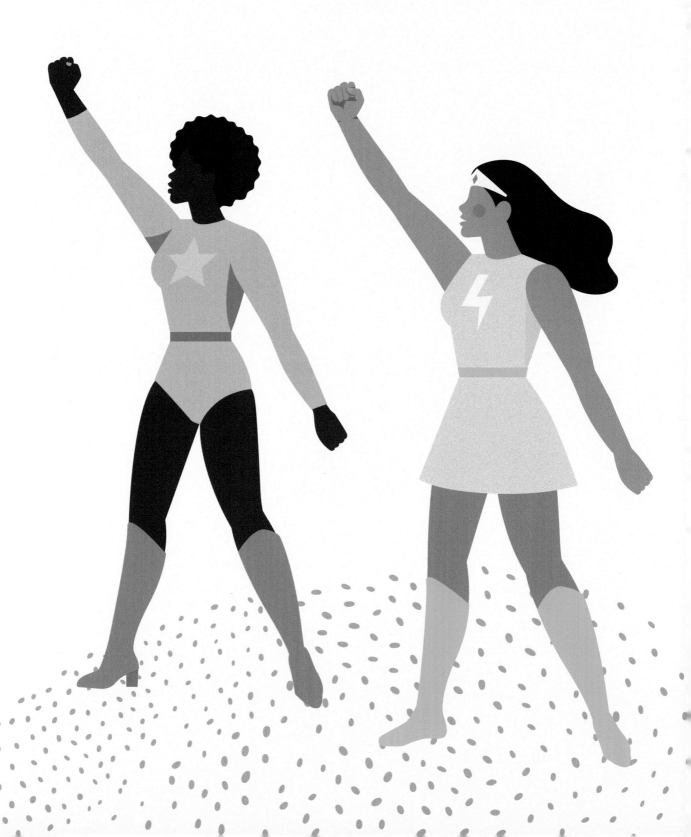

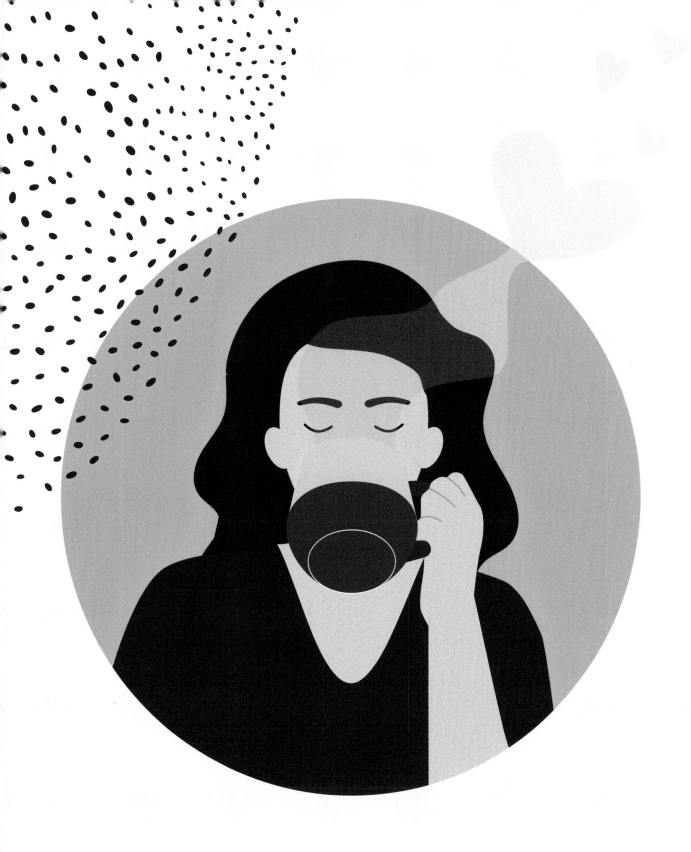

Power Foods/Drinks

It's necessary to recognise which foods and drinks bring you joy, to learn to relish them, and to regularly bring them into your diet. These aren't the things you crave because of a sugar low, or because they're your go-to comfort foods. Your Power Foods/Drinks are the things that you enjoy eating because they make you feel good in the moment and afterwards. They make you smile when you're eating them, they digest easily in your system, energise you, and make you feel like you did something self-loving by consuming them.

I'm not a trained nutritionist but I've been on a million different diets - from raw vegan to blood type (O+) meat eating - and discovered that if I got quiet, listened, and had a more curious relationship with food instead of a restrictive one I could clearly hear what my body wanted. I suggest that you do the same and understand that it may take a while to really pinpoint what works best for you. Take some time to experiment with different foods, smoothies, salads and notice how you feel before, during, and after you eat them especially if you're preparing them yourself. Your Power Foods/Drinks will make you grin while you're cooking them, make you pause as you chew your first bite, and make you feel great afterwards.

One of my favourites is my first cup of coffee of the day. I relish it, I smile at it, hold it with both hands as if it were precious gold, and I talk to it! I tell it how delicious it is and I say "Thank you" aloud.

Each of the practices above are meant to bring you into a sense of feeling fantastic and empowered. When you need to go full Superhero, try combining all of them. Organise a get together with a friend or small group of friends with whom there's a high level of mutual trust and support. Take turns running through the songs in your Power Playlists, wear your Power/Superhero Costumes, enjoy your Power Foods and Drinks, and dance like there's no tomorrow!

If your group feels really safe together, play a game where you express what you love and admire about each person, giving everyone a turn to go around the room. Then do some journaling about how it made you feel to hear words of admiration, and also how it might have triggered you. Share thoughts from your journaling and have the others offer support to reaffirm the positive and to redirect negative beliefs.

What's most essential about the Superhero exercises is that you notice the elevated emotions and lean into them in order to cultivate higher vibrations. Then when the negative loop rears its ugly head (and it will, purely out of efficiency), you are equipped with new tools: Take a pause, redirect your thoughts, and utilise one or more of your Superhero exercises. Imprint the sensation you want to have and let the old one go. Now, this will be challenging at first. Your limbic system will try to tell you "but we've had the old belief for a long time. It's familiar. This new positive feeling takes time and energy". Your limbic system may even get grumpy and act like a disgruntled toddler at times. This is where you pause and ask yourself:"who do I want to be at this moment?". In the beginning, the old belief systems will win out more often than you'd like, but keep at it. The power is in the noticing when negative thoughts creep up. Replace the old beliefs with the ENERGY of the new belief - not just a thought. When you keep replacing it with the new positive feeling, eventually that becomes part of the loop, creating your new normal.

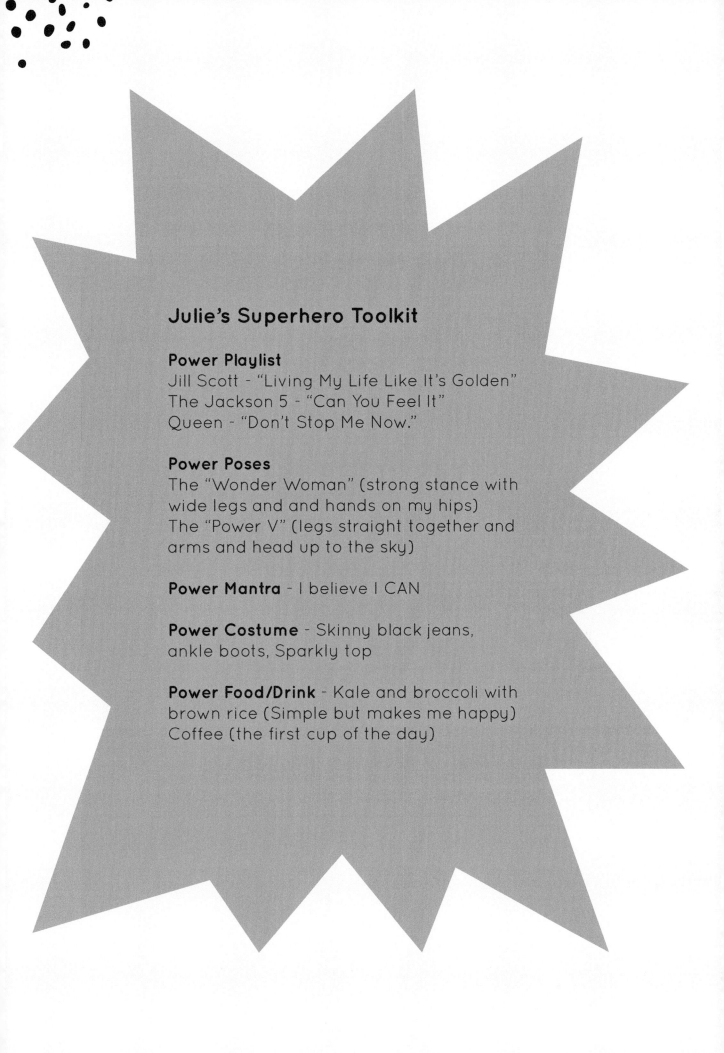

Julie's Superhero Toolkit

Power Playlist
Jill Scott - "Living My Life Like It's Golden"
The Jackson 5 - "Can You Feel It"
Queen - "Don't Stop Me Now."

Power Poses
The "Wonder Woman" (strong stance with wide legs and and hands on my hips)
The "Power V" (legs straight together and arms and head up to the sky)

Power Mantra - I believe I CAN

Power Costume - Skinny black jeans, ankle boots, Sparkly top

Power Food/Drink - Kale and broccoli with brown rice (Simple but makes me happy)
Coffee (the first cup of the day)

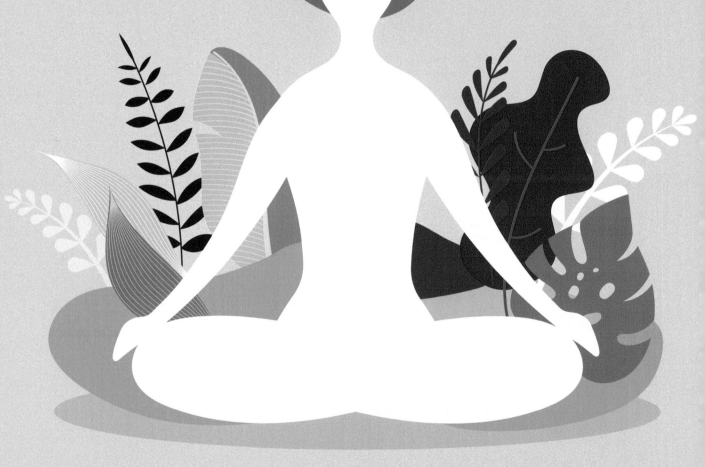

"We ask ourselves, who am I to be brilliant, gorgeous, talented, fabulous? Actually, who are you not to be? You are a child of God. Your playing small does not serve the world. There is nothing enlightened about shrinking so that other people won't feel insecure around you."

Marianne Williamson

2. Creative empowerment

The word "creativity" can make some people immediately break out into a rash. As you have discovered in the Pillars of Transformation, our belief systems sometimes get us out of sync with our true nature. As Marianne Williamson has said, we are all creative beings. Being creative is our true nature. The sad truth is that we are usually raised to believe that some people are talented and the rest of us should "stick to our day jobs." Or perhaps your experience was the opposite. You might have had a talent for piano or singing or art, and were told to diligently master your craft with strict discipline until it was no longer fun. And all of this concentration in one area might have come at the expense of sacrificing other creative endeavours.

Either way, as human beings we are naturally creative. We are creating all the time whether we realise it or not. Talent is not just reserved for the fortunate few; we all have a talent and usually more than one. They're just often hidden by self-doubt or disregarded because we don't see the inherent creativity in so many of our actions.

I have friends who swear they have no creative talent. Then I get invited over for dinner to discover they are the kind of people who can whip up an amazing meal in under an hour. They confess that they are passionate about cooking and experimenting with recipes and flavours, and yet don't recognise that this is an art. It's expressive, it's enjoyable for them, and it makes others happy too. How wonderful and creative!

On the flip side, I have a friend who works in multi-million dollar finance and loves her job because she sees the creativity and expression in it every day. She doesn't see money as a means to an end, she sees it as energy that she can move and use as a tool to explore more possibilities. She finds it unfortunate that many finance investors stick to rigid formulas, usually as an outward expression of their need for control, while she uses her hippie-fied viewpoint to have a more fluid and creative relationship with money. Needless to say, she is extremely successful.

The above scenarios are just two small examples of what creativity can be. Dancing, singing, visual art, and music usually come to mind when we think about creative outlets, but even these don't necessarily require talent in order to enjoy the process of creativity. I know wonderful singing teachers who can get an entire room of novices to find their voices and make lovely music together, and art teachers who can elicit something beautiful from people who have picked up a paint brush for the first time. As we dive into this next section, let's set aside our old parameters about creativity and embrace the idea that what we are really exploring is self-expression. And this is why we may have hesitation. When we express ourselves - our ideas, our thoughts, and our creative endeavours - we risk judgement. It becomes personal and it's easier to hide rather than expose ourselves to potential embarrassment or shame. This is why this section is titled Creative Empowerment. When we understand the layers that may be covering up our creativity and let go of judgement, either from ourselves or from others, then we can delve into the unknown and become empowered by the possibilities. We can learn to change our dialogue from "I'm not very good at art/singing/music/creating" to "I'm willing to try anything and see where the process takes me".

In this section we will cover why creativity is important for everyone and how it is linked to our deep transformation. We'll look at our relationship with vulnerability and how to hold it as a sacred power. And we'll learn to tame our inner critic so that we embrace curiosity over judgement. Once we get to grips with these concepts, we'll go through several exercises to flex our creativity muscles and bring self-expression into our everyday lives.

Why Creativity Is Important

A great deal of research has been done over the past few decades about creativity and how it affects our wellbeing, problem-solving skills, productivity, and self-awareness. It has become evident that the less we are encouraged to engage in creative activities, the more fear we have around expressing ourselves in our own unique ways. There is a tendency to stick to the status quo and avoid being innovative or having differing opinions. In fact, with children now participating in fewer creative outlets at school (often due to budget cuts), they're more hesitant to even attempt self-expression, resulting in a multitude of issues concerning a lack of self-confidence that show up later in their teen and young adult years.

For example, Anne Pyburn Craig notes in her article *Creative Development* in *Early Childhood:* "Solid scientific research indicates that encouraging creativity, not just by exposure to art and music during the foundational years before 5, but by encouraging creative approaches to problem-solving, communication and everyday activities, enhances happiness and life satisfaction in a lasting way"[2].

Additionally, many recent studies have highlighted the critical importance for adults to play, learn something new, and explore creative outlets (just for fun as opposed to mastering them) in order to create new neural pathways and enhance cognitive capabilities. An article on Americannurse.com states:

"Most of the studies agree that engagement in the arts decreases depressive symptoms, increases positive emotions, reduces stress, and in some cases, improves immune system functioning."

"Other studies found that creative works and exposure to the arts can impact conditions like Parkinson's disease and some forms of dementia and cancer. Creative wellness is good for your intellectual wellness, too. A study by the Mayo Clinic found that people who engage in activities like painting, drawing, sculpting, and crafts (woodworking, pottery, ceramics, quilting) in middle-age and older may delay cognitive decline"[3].

Whether you're looking to be creatively inspired in your favourite art form or just tune into your own wellbeing, the research overwhelmingly shows that engaging in creative endeavours is just as necessary as learning how to read and write. It plays a crucial role in how we find our way in the world.

Years ago, I enrolled in a basic drawing class at my local college just to try something different that didn't involve movement or performing (my life's work up until that point). It was recommended that we read a book by Betty Edwards called *Drawing on the Right Side of the Brain*. That book blew me away by its explanation of how we mainly focus on the functions of the left side of the brain, especially now that we live in a digital age. Edwards states that activating the right side of the brain is extremely valuable in that:

"The ability to draw on the strengths of the right hemisphere can serve as an antidote to the increasing left-brain emphasis in American life - the worship of all that is linear, analytic, digital, etc...We power up the brain's plasticity when learning new skills that utilize the right hemisphere of the brain".

That drawing class helped me to view the world with different perspectives by activating the right side of my brain, and I discovered that I'm pretty damn good artist - which was a pleasant surprise!

We are also using the right side of our brain when we are in a meditative state, as this side doesn't calculate time or space. As we delve into our process of Creative Empowerment, keep in mind that there is so much more going on than trying to create a painting, song, dance, etc. We're creating new neural pathways and shifting our perception which is vital for our personal transformation.

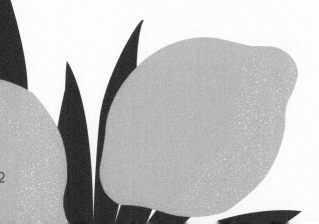

1. Vulnerability is the key to creativity

Vulnerability is probably something that we spend a majority of our lives trying to avoid. It's uncomfortable. It can give us the "naked in a room full of clothed people" sensation. Any scenario where we feel vulnerable always hits deeply in the gut. Our whole body gets involved. Even just recollecting a time when we found ourselves in a vulnerable situation is enough to get our hearts racing, our palms sweating, and our stomachs clenching up.

Just for fun, see how you feel when reading each of the following scenarios:

- Telling someone you love them for the first time

- A job interview or audition

- Having to relay news that you know the other person doesn't want to hear

- Receiving criticism, even if it's delivered in a compassionate and constructive way

- Presenting something you've created

Now consider this: what happens when you witness someone else being vulnerable? Most likely you'll admire their strength and courage to meet the situation head-on and with grace. You'll understand that this person is in acceptance of the unknown and is still willing to put themselves out there. It's inspiring and reassuring to watch, right? That's because there is power in our vulnerability.

"When we stop worrying about what others might think and truly allow ourselves to be expressive, the door to our creative powers opens up and welcomes us in."

— Julie Martin

Vulnerability is vital to our creativity, as our ability to create relies on our honesty and authenticity to ourselves. But we need to drop our armour to get to that place. So many of us keep our creative endeavours or our passionate ideas secret from others for fear of being judged, ridiculed, or shamed.

I see this a lot in the yoga world. Many teachers are actually afraid to teach according to what feels genuine to them, instead delivering a class based on what they think their students want. Some teachers have told me how much they love my work - the creative sequences and embodiment workshops - but they could never do that themselves. They worry that their students won't like it, or it will go against the studio's tradition or the lineage in which they were taught. It takes a lot of courage to show up and teach what you believe in and not worry about the naysayers.

I'll tell you this, when you do show up as your genuine self you'll feel amazing! And the bonus is that if it feels authentic to you, then it will feel authentic to your students too. Because it's coming from a place of truth - your truth.

There is a current creativity deficit in many industries worldwide because so many work environments don't encourage vulnerability. They reward being tough, working hard, and moving along with the status quo. Exhaustion has become a status symbol.There is no room for people to speak up and make suggestions about new ideas or concepts for fear of being shot down. And yet, without creativity, we have no way to move forward. Where would we be as a culture without new ways of communicating, designing, or developments in everything from the medical sector to how we clean our clothes? We'd probably be stuck in the caveman era merely surviving.

Like everything else, vulnerability is a state-of-being that we can learn to sink into so that it becomes more and more comfortable for us. We can decide that each moment that makes us feel vulnerable is an opportunity to grow and evolve. This is not only necessary for developing our own self-confidence, but also it frees up our ability to be creative with possibilities that we might have shied away from before.

I've mainly uncovered my own relationship with vulnerability through Brené Brown's work. In her book Daring Greatly she opens with the following quote by Theodore Roosevelt (the 26th President of the United States) from his 1910 speech *Citizenship in a Republic*:

"It is not the critic who counts; not the man who points out how the strong man stumbles, or where the doer of deeds could have done them better. The credit belongs to the man who is actually in the arena, whose face is marred by dust and sweat and blood; who strives valiantly; who errs, who comes short again and again, because there is no effort without error and shortcoming; but who does actually strive to do the deeds; who knows great enthusiasms, the great devotions; who spends himself in a worthy cause; who at the best knows in the end the triumph of high achievement, and who at the worst, if he fails, at least fails while daring greatly, so that his place shall never be with those cold and timid souls who neither know victory nor defeat."

What I love about this quote and Brené Brown's work is that the concept of being vulnerable gets turned around and we learn to embrace our ability to "dare greatly." For me, the idea of "daring greatly" feels more like rising to a challenge to navigate through something that makes me feel vulnerable, and the more that I do it the more comfortable I become. For example, you might feel nervous talking in front of a group of people (most people do), but once you've done it a few times and survived you realise it gets easier each time. It's more than okay to feel vulnerable, it's actually part of the process. From there, we grow.

EXERCISES

Vulnerability is such an individual thing. I can comfortably speak in front of large groups, I've traveled the world on my own, and have learned how to gracefully handle difficult and awkward conversations. However, if you asked me to walk across a beach in just a bikini, strike up a conversation with a handsome man, or ask me to bring a dish to a potluck, I will start quaking at the knees and my heart will pound out of my chest.
The following exercises will help you assess your own vulnerability triggers and then take steps to move through them *constructively*. We've all probably heard the phrase "Do something every day that scares you".
I like the sentiment but I always want to make sure it's part of my individual growth. I'm afraid of jumping into a cold ocean, but I could do it, jump back out, and it wouldn't really help me to start my own business or write a novel. With these exercises, you'll explore actions that move you toward your development and creativity by doing things that you really want to do but may have been afraid to attempt.

The Lists

The Shine List
As with our gratitude work in the first section, it's great to start with things that we have a positive relationship with: creative endeavours and talents that we already feel confident about. One of mine is my ability to create well-constructed yoga and movement sequences that are unique to my way of teaching. Even when I get screwed up or realise I haven't quite thought something through all the way, I know that I can remedy any issues quickly and creatively.

Now it's your turn. On the following spread you'll find a worksheet with two columns.

THE LEFT COLUMN - Where you already shine
On the left column labelled "Where I shine" write 5-10 things that you know you're good at. It's not just about the big things so consider small talents and skills too. Remember that many things we do involve some kind of creative thinking. If you're already scratching your head, then ask a trusted family member or friend. We often can't see our inherent talents when they are things we do simply because we love them.

THE RIGHT COLUMN - How it makes you feel
Review each of your talents one at a time. Close your eyes and breathe the sensation. Ask yourself:"Is this talent part of who I am or is it cultivated from years of practice? How does it make me feel about myself? How does it serve me out in the world?". On the right column labelled "How it makes me feel" write a short sentence based on the questions above and whatever else pops into your mind.

Once you've finished that worksheet, remember to pat yourself on the back. You ARE creative and talented. These exercises are really about getting beyond our judgement filters.

The Boost List
The next part of The Lists involves exploring our vulnerability triggers, our fears around them, and how to mitigate our self-doubt. Here I will confess my own vulnerability triggers around putting together this workbook. I thought; *"Oh no, I'm afraid this is going to turn into a book about spirituality. Who am I to write about that? I'm not a guru, a shaman, or a priest. What if I make a fool of myself?"*. Then I thought about all of the different things I have studied in earnest, the practices that I've adopted in my own spiritual journey, and the positive comments from my students over the years. I realised that I've already been doing extensive spiritual development work for quite some time and now I'm just consolidating my experiences into this workbook!

On the following spread you'll find a worksheet with three columns.

THE LEFT COLUMN - What you'd like to try
In the column labelled "What I'd like to try" list 5-10 things you've been wanting to do but have stopped yourself. Your list can include big things like changing careers, performing in public, or starting your own business, and seemingly small things like baking a speciality cake, taking up salsa dancing, dusting off your sewing machine and making something. Complete this list by filling out the column vertically (top to bottom).

THE MIDDLE COLUMN - The fear dump
Review the first item you listed in the left column. In the middle column labelled "The fear dump" write one or two reasons why the idea of doing this thing brings up fear for you. Does it trigger perceived disapproval from a loved one or close friend? Are you afraid you won't be good at it? Are you afraid you will be good at it? Are you afraid it will bring up new insights about yourself you're not ready to address?

THE RIGHT COLUMN- What would your best friend say
In the right column labelled "Your best friend's comment" imagine what your best friend would say to you if you expressed your fear to them. Write that down. Go ahead and utilise your friend's word choices, funny sayings, and even their f-bombs if that's how they speak. Read your "best friend's" words aloud and feel that sensation.

Repeat Steps 1 - 3 for each item on your list.
Use both the Shine and Boost list as a reflection tool. In moments of doubt remind yourself what you're already good at and what your best friend would say to your fears.

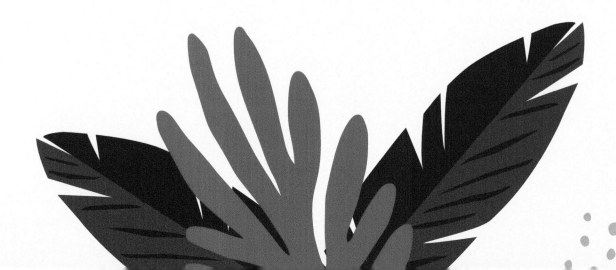

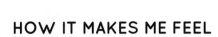

WHERE I SHINE

HOW IT MAKES ME FEEL

WHAT I'D LIKE TO TRY	THE FEAR DUMP	WHAT MY BEST FRIEND WOULD SAY

Take That (Mini) Step!

Now that you've identified 5-10 things you'd like to try, you can begin to venture into your vulnerability zone by learning something about your new endeavour before taking a giant leap. While some things will be easier to jump into than others, like Zumba as a way to pave the way into salsa dancing, remember that these mini steps can be used as emotional stepping stones. Getting vulnerable with the smaller aspects of our dreams allows us to feel our way through them and start accumulating the building blocks of courage.

Review the things on your Boost List and circle the one that seems most appealing to you right now. This is another "trust your gut" moment. Or close your eyes, swirl the paper around, and randomly put your finger on one of them.

Take a mico-action toward your mini step. Research options to find a class, a mentor, a tutorial, companies and/or universities that interest you, opportunities for an internship, a fellowship, a scholarship, or people to schedule an informational interview with. This is about exploring the possibilities.

Ask a very trusted person to be your Accountability Buddy. Your Accountability Buddy is the person with whom you're going to check in with regarding your progress every little step of the way. Now take the next indicated mico-action, which could be signing up for a class, sending an email, filling out an application. Check in with your Accountability Buddy via text or a short call *before and after* hitting send on the computer, having that phone conversation, or clicking the confirm button, etc. Your Accountability Buddy might even want to support you further by taking a class with you, reviewing your writing, or tasting that new specialty cake you're trying out. Let them see your progress and share in your moments of vulnerability.

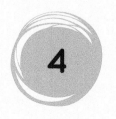

Take that mini-step with complete curiosity for the process. Notice how you feel in the beginning. And as you progress, what is evolving with your self-talk? Keep checking in with your Accountability Buddy. You may discover the joy of doing things without needing them to be perfect or even complete.

Perhaps you start a class in something, dabble in it for a while, and realise it's not too scary anymore and be done with it. That's a great result. We start off anxious and hesitant, we meet our vulnerability and then realise we can do something we thought we couldn't. Being in a balanced relationship with vulnerability is never about "getting over it". It's about knowing we'll be OK whatever the outcome. But we try, we take those first baby steps. We get in the arena. We "dare greatly".

"Courage is not the absence of fear, but rather the judgement that something else is more important than fear."

Ambrose Redmoon

Vulnerability Meditation

This meditation is about connecting to what makes us feel safe and stable. When we have a sense of that, we can trust that the Universe has our back. We can step our toes into the unknown feeling supported. This is a great meditation to do before taking those first mini steps in order to ground ourselves in our courage. Either read through the instructions below or just play the video where I guide you through.

Watch video number 4: "Meditation-Vulnerability"

Find a comfortable place to sit and take a moment to notice how your body feels in this position. Notice your breath as it is, no need to change it. Do a body scan from bottom to top and sense where there may be tension and ask your body to release it. Don't judge it if you have a difficult time releasing this tension. We're just asking first.

Take a moment to swallow to relax your jaw and throat. Then bring your awareness down to your sit bones. Whether you're on a chair or sitting on the floor, become aware of how they are connected to the ground. Notice the sensation that the ground gives you. Do you feel supported? Does this support allow you to relax in your pelvis a bit more? Can you drop your breath into your belly? Keep your awareness with your breath for 10 rounds, while noticing the sensations around your pelvis, thighs, sit bones and lower back.

- Ask your inner voice or higher power: "Am I safe? Am I supported?". Just let the answer come in whatever form it encompasses.

- If you hear a "No" just note that it's only your limbic system doing its auto-loop and keep breathing until you feel the sensation of being safe and supported.

- Visualise yourself doing one of the things on your Boost List.

- Cultivate the sensation of being comfortable doing that thing that makes you feel vulnerable.

- Now bring in the sounds, smells, and sights that would be around you in this triumphant moment.

- If you start to feel anxious, just go back to the questions: "Am I safe? Am I supported?"

- Get back to that scenario of doing the thing from your list, and the sensation of trust in yourself

- Sit with this sensation as long as you can.

Remember, when you find yourself in a spacious moment you are perceiving from the right side or your brain where there is no analysis or calculation of time. You also lose you negative self-talk in this space so it's crucial to make that 'imprint' of being courageous onto your cells. My hope is that the above vulnerability exercises will help you to feel more comfortable in any challenging situation. The key to accessing your creative power lies in understanding that the first few attempts at anything new can be frightening, stir up self-doubt, and send you running to 'safety' even if it means losing out on something you think you might love doing. By continuing to strengthen your courage and constructively moving through vulnerable situations - step by mini step - will you be expanding your confidence and creativity at the same time.

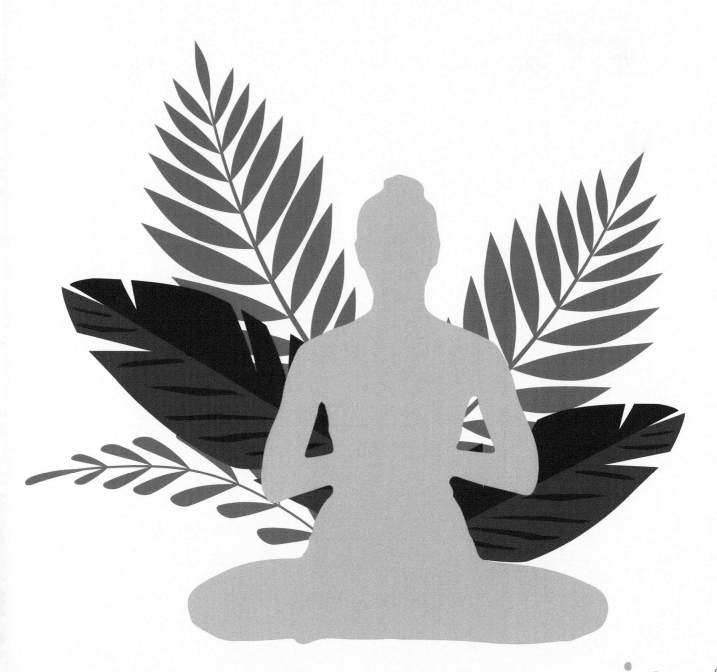

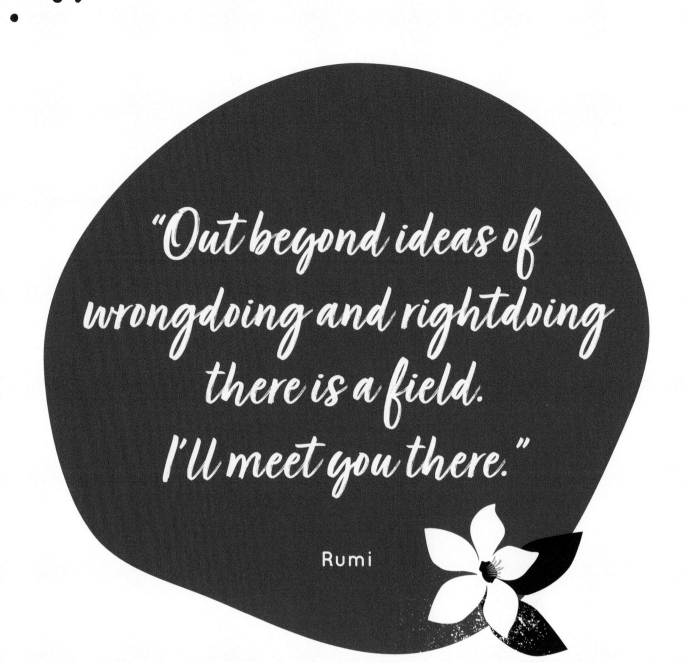

"Out beyond ideas of wrongdoing and rightdoing there is a field. I'll meet you there."

Rumi

2. The inner critic

I mentor and coach a lot of yoga teachers worldwide. I deeply enjoy working with people who are ready to nurture their talent and skills in an effort to further their students' relationships with movement, meditation, and wellbeing. While my own students come from many different demographics and cultures there is one constant that I see in almost every single person: imposter syndrome.

It happens to everyone at some point. Even myself. I've been teaching and refining my skills for over 30 years and yet, I can still catch myself before a workshop thinking: "I'm not sure I know what I'm talking about" and "who's going to be interested in listening anyway?". Crazy, huh? But I've learned to use this inner critic in a positive and productive way. This is why all the work that we've done together throughout the previous sections is so significant. It lays the foundation for understanding the difference between our inner guide or higher power and our limiting belief systems and unfounded fears.

When we see imposter syndrome running towards us with arms wide open ready to squeeze the life out of our confidence, we can learn to put our hands up and say "Stop! In the name of love". Corny, I know but it's actually true. When we feel that inner critic giving us the list of reasons why we're crap at something we can flip the criticism on its head through self-compassion. Our critic can be our friend when it becomes a check-in for our own personal standards.

When the inner critic arrives, what if instead of giving it a microphone we gave ourselves a loving deep breath and paused to ask ourselves some compassionate questions?

Let's take the example of my getting ready for a workshop. When I hear the negative voices creep up, usually about an hour before start time, I pause and ask: "Have you spent the last months researching what you're talking about today? - Yes. If you had to sit down and explain all of these concepts to your best friend would they find it interesting? - Yes. Have these students signed up because they like your work? - Yes. Do you have 30 years of experience? - Yes." And so on.

This process gives me the bigger picture about myself. It reminds me that I hold myself to high standards. It's OK to have an inner critic, but I need to counter it with questions that challenge any self-doubt. If I'm met with uncertainty then I know I need to do more preparation or take a different approach, but I don't have to limit my work or creativity because a crazy voice in my head says, "You're not good enough". My reply is: "Prove it".

When we hold onto ideas of right or wrong during our creative explorations, we remain in judgement; judgement of ourselves and fear about how others may judge us. This often spawns creative paralysis. By moving beyond the notions of a "right" and "wrong" way in any area we learn to understand, describe, and associate things with how we feel in the process as opposed to struggling for "success" or avoiding "failure" (according to some standard that might not even be our own).

Imagine there was no "right" and "wrong" way to do something; there is just your way in this moment. Sometimes it will look like a mess, sometimes it will make sense, but neither outcome is wrong or bad. Remember the old adage: "What would you do if you know you couldn't fail?". Well, that's just it: you can't fail. Failure is a perception based on what someone else told you was right. Remove the rules and regulations and then you can remove the fear of getting it wrong.

EXERCISES

Push The Pause Button

As I've described above, we can convert the inner critic into being an ally for personal accountability. If we're about to embark on a creative journey that makes us feel anxious and uncertain, it's highly likely that our inner critic is talking to us loudly and incessantly. However, we can take stock of reality in this moment and do so by pausing and asking ourselves some good questions.

If you've been wanting to take an art or dance class but you're nervous you'll be bad at it, ask some questions before surrendering to the voice of the inner critic:

Does it matter if I'm good or bad as long as I enjoy it?
How will I know if I really like (singing/cooking/sewing) if I don't try it?
What is the worst thing that can happen if I go ahead and write a book or design a hat?

If it's a something in your usual realm of work/career and your imposter syndrome regularly sneaks in, ask yourself check-in questions:

Have I done my research?
Is this the first time I'm doing this? (If Yes then it's OK to make mistakes. If No then maybe you've got this!)
Have I completed my tasks to a standard I feel comfortable with?
Do other people in my field also feel nervous about doing/ presenting this? (The answer is always Yes, so remember you're in good company as we all have self-doubt!)

If what you're experimenting with is planting seeds for your bigger dreams and ideas, ask this one question:

If I never attempt this thing, how will I feel about it at the end of my life?

Remember the goal here isn't to totally "slay the beast" (i.e. your inner critic), because it's your inner critic that holds you to your own high standards. You only need to be just slightly more committed to taking a mini step toward your goal than you are to listening to your inner critic. To paraphrase the quote by Theordore Roosevent, you have to at least get in the arena. We are then in a process of growth that can only lead to confidence, even if we get it wrong a few times.

Journaling

These exercises are about consciously choosing curiosity over judgement by noticing the voice of the inner critic and turning it around. Let's get rid of our right vs wrong/good vs bad dialogue and ask: *"What if everything I did was just about learning, exploring, and being open to what evolves from the process?"*.

Journaling Part 1: Coal into diamonds

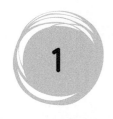
The Event
Think about moments in your past where it seemed like you had made a horrible mistake or a bad decision, or just felt like you were floundering. For example, quitting a job, moving house or starting a project that didn't work, etc. List 3-5 of these seemingly bad decisions/moments.

The Inner Critic
Go through each event from your list and write 1-2 sentences on how you felt at that time. What was the self-talk?

The Outcome
Now write a paragraph (4-6 sentences) about the eventual outcome of each event and the things you learned about yourself. How did your story evolve afterwards?

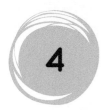
Inspired Growth
Write a few sentences about how this experience inspired growth that you have integrated into your life. What did you learn about yourself that made a deep connection?

Example:

Event - When I submitted an original short story to a theater company.

Inner Critic - You've never done this before, you don't know what you're doing, they're going to hate it and the story is very personal so it will be a double personal rejection.

Outcome - The story was rejected by the theater company and I was depressed for days. But half a year later one of the readers passed it onto his film producer wife. She thought that it would make a better short film and optioned my story for that instead. This resulted in a wider audience viewing my story and I've subsequently been asked to write more for film production.

Inspired Growth - I remind myself daily that I believe in myself regardless of what the outcomes might be, and that it's more important that I show up for my creative self. I do the work and the Universe creates the outcome. I'm open to all possibilities.

Journaling Part 2: The "what ifs?"'"

Hopefully the Coal into diamonds journaling exercise helped shed some light on how your choices or just change in circumstances assisted in some way with your personal development and you gained confidence in where you are at this moment. Now we're going to engage in a similar exercise using recent events.

Event
List 1-3 things that you are currently working on. A new project or goal or current aspects of a job you are trying to improve. Maybe it's something you've got on the right side of your Gratitude Journal.

Inner Critic
Go through each thing from your list and write 2-3 sentences about what your inner critic is saying. What is your hesitation or perceived obstacles?

What If's
For each thing on your list write a few sentences that put a spin on them and open up the possibilities using "What if...?" statements (see example below)

Example:

Event - I'm creating my own online course.

Inner critic - I'm not good enough. Other teachers have similar content so why would somebody do my course? Even if they do my course they're not going to like it.

What if's - What if I reach even one person and my course has a huge impact on them? What if the next time I offer the course it sells out? What if someone does my course and invites me to teach it in person? What if I get asked to do a TED Talk as a result of the popularity of my course?

It doesn't matter if it sounds 'fantastical' because we honestly don't know what our long term outcomes will be. Only time can tell. So if we dedicate ourselves to our process and creative endeavours and are open to possibilities we can keep our inner critic in check.

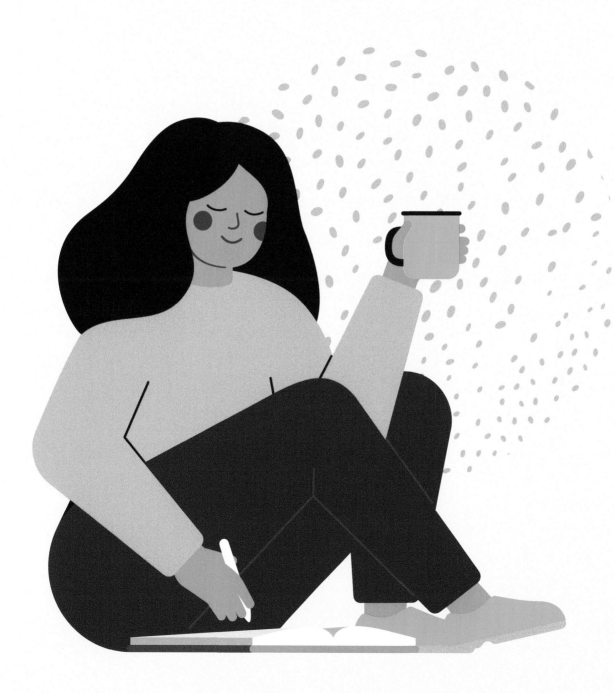

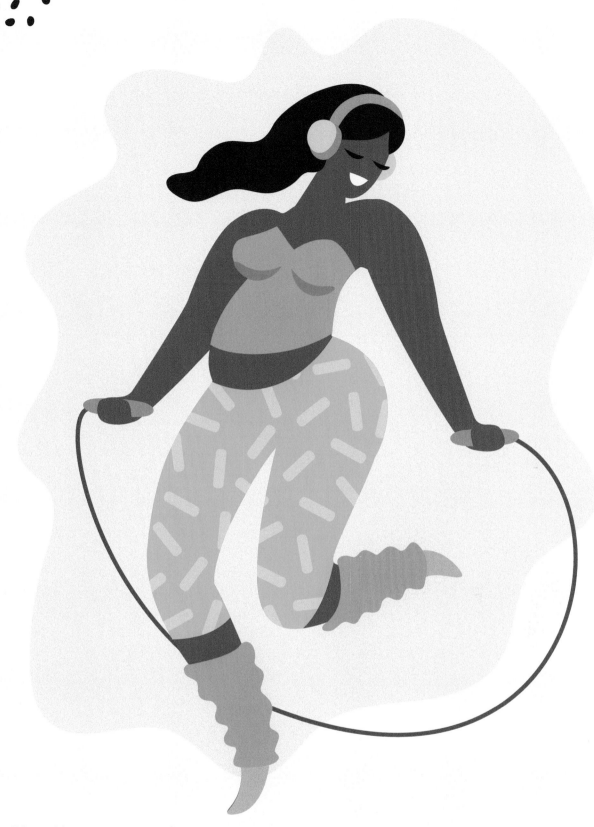

3. Playtime everyday

After we have forged a relationship with our vulnerability and understand how to turn down the volume on our inner critic it's PLAYTIME! Playing and creativity go hand in hand. Remember those D.O.S.E. hormones (dopamine, oxytocin, serotonin and endorphins) discussed in the Superhero section? These mood-boosting, immune system-bolstering, energizing hormones get released when we're having fun "just playing around". This surge allows us to connect with what we are passionate about because it becomes less self-critical and more exploratory. Some of the best ideas can come to us when we're scribbling, dabbling in something, or physically playing with friends and family, etc. In fact, many inventions emerged out of playful curiosity rather than the old adage of "Necessity is the mother of invention".

While it seems like play is only acceptable for children, and not something for adults, the research shows that play is vitally important at any age. Just look up articles, books and podcasts on the importance of adult play and you'll be busy for days with all the information that is out there. Here's just one tidbit from a paper published in *Psychology Today*:

"It (play) may in fact be the highest expression of our humanity, both imitating and advancing the evolutionary process. Play appears to allow our brains to exercise their very flexibility, to maintain and even perhaps renew the neural connections that embody our human potential to adapt, to meet any possible set of environmental conditions"[4].

Given the rapid speed with which we are now taking in information and increasing our productivity in the workplace, it's no surprise that more and more of us are searching for a playful outlet as a counterbalance. Notice the number of adult colouring books on the shelves these days? And the market for video games, which used to be exclusive to teenage boys, now targets adults as well by touting them as stress relievers and brain exercisers.

If we lose our sense of play and creativity we lose the ability to create new neural pathways. Also, as different parts of the brain become less active, we become fearful of the idea of doing or learning something new. So it's not just self-judgement kicking in, it's that we actually lose the software to be creative. The saying "You can't teach an old dog new tricks" is valid because the dog wasn't encouraged to keep playing and learning new tricks in the first place, not because he got old.

EXERCISES

So let's play! Several different options are offered below. A few of them are based on Stuart Brown's work (See Resources), and I've added some of my own favourites. It's not expected that you do all of them. Choose one or two that grab you. And remember, if any of the suggestions begin to wake up your inner critic or perfectionist, try something else. Don't worry about getting things right when you're playing. On the other hand, you may end up being really good at some of your playtime activities, and that's OK too. Just keep in mind that the only goal here is finding your joy.

Different types of play:

Storytelling

We all have an internal narrative and a natural instinct for storytelling. It's often how our brain processes information and how we retell it to others. It's great if you've got a captive audience of children or others to make up stories with together. Or you can make this into a group activity on "digital free days" (which are necessary). Pick a topic and have everyone create a little story to share. Or you can play the game where one person starts off with a sentence and you go around the room as each individual adds the next sentence to the story. Journaling your stories is a great non-social option. No one needs to read your journal, but it's imperative that your stories, thoughts, and ideas have a place to be expressed. I suggest checking out *The Artist's Way* by Julia Cameron for the Morning Pages exercise (See Resources).

Body Play

Moving the body just for fun by dancing, wiggling, or shimmying around to your favourite tunes can be an incredible release. So is playing physical games or sports, specifically if it's combined with socialising. For example, meeting up with a friend once a week to play tennis and then have lunch together is not only beneficial for our physical well being, but our brains love it when we have a social connection with our playtime. Physical play with a pet is another excellent endorphin stimulator. Many studies have shown that elderly people who have a pet, particularly a dog, have a stronger immune system and better mental health than those who don't. I've made a video as part of this course where we will play and explore movement around a few different themes.

Watch video number 5: "Fun Movement Play"

Object Play

This can include activities like crafting, collaging, working with clay or playdough, or building something even if it's with a toy like Lego. The brain revels in it when we feel our experience through our hands.

Pretending and Imagination

Our imaginative scenarios are really powerful creative tools. Theatre and drama classes are perfect for this because we can play a role without the pressure to perform (although that might happen too). Additionally, going to fun places that are usually reserved for children - like an amusement park, petting zoo, or miniature golf - are wonderful ways to play and be imaginative. My sister used to work at Disneyland in Anaheim, California. She said sometimes the parents appeared to be having more fun than the children when they allowed themselves to relax and surrender to the make-believe element.

Spectator Play

When we're watching others engage in a sport, performance, or game it's easy to get emotionally involved and feel the rush as if we were the ones doing the activity. This is why watching a live sporting event, a theatre production, a comedy show, or a concert with a group of friends is a really uplifting activity, because it immerses us in a sense of fun, wonder, awe, or suspense. Ideally it will be something that you'll enjoy talking about days after to prolong the effect of the experience.

The Space Out

This is one of my own, I do it often, and was initially surprised that other people don't regularly do this. I take some "space out" time almost every day, usually after I've been working on the computer or finished teaching a class. I like to lay down on the floor and just let my mind wander. It's never critical thinking or toggling between past and future events; it's just letting my thoughts meander wherever they want to go. If I'm near a window, I'll notice the sky or trees outside or listen to the surrounding noises.

By doing this for many years, I've realised how much inspiration I derive from these moments. I'm not really thinking about anything and then suddenly a thought pops into my head about a new project or a solution to an old problem. Sometimes I'm only 10 minutes into my "space out" time and I get loads of ideas, and other times I lay there for half an hour and nothing substantial arises. Many people might think this is just wasting time; on the contrary, it's giving your nervous system and your prefrontal cortex a complete break. Even if nothing comes up for me, I get up and get back to my work with a fresh mind.

Whatever and however you decide to play, the crucial thing is that you're not looking for an outcome that has a judgement or comparison attached to it. We want our play to be something that is not attached to failure or success. Let go of judgement and instead get excited that you're working parts of your brain to form new neural pathways of thought and expression, thus opening a doorway to expanded possibilities.

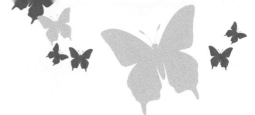

4. Vision boards and movies

Vision boards may have started as a cutesy crafting activity, but now evidence shows that there is significant power in regularly seeing a vision of your future self. While many of you may already be familiar with vision boards, and perhaps have even made a few, let's review what a vision board is really about. Just how the Gratitude Journal is a written testament to what you're working to manifest, a vision board creates a visual image of that future. What I really relish about working with vision boards is that it's a fully immersive creative process. We allow our vision to come to life as a tangible expression of ourselves.

Specifically, a vision board is a collage of pictures from magazines, books, actual photos, and anything else that captures a sense of how you want to feel in your life. As with your Gratitude Journal the goal is to find images that cultivate the sensations around what you are manifesting. However, this is where using magazines can get a bit difficult because they're designed to sell us stuff.

Let's take an example: I want to have a healthy and joyous relationship with my body just as it is. If I choose a photo of a woman in a bikini with a great body sitting on a beach, that might not create the sensation I'm after. In fact, it may even have the opposite effect and invoke a sense of dissatisfaction because I don't have the same body as the model. A better image would be one of someone who looks like they are enjoying life and celebrating who they are. Yes, this is challenging with most fashion magazines, but there are options out there like *O Magazine* and others, that focus on holistic wellbeing and are not so fixated on selling us an unrealistic ideal.

Personally I love collecting images and keeping them in a box until I'm in the mood to make a vision board. The curiosity that arises as I sift through the images becomes therapeutic. Using my hands, cutting and pasting, and often adding texture with glitter or feathers or other things I've gathered keeps my mind occupied and fully relaxed. When it's finished, I suggest posting your vision board at your desk, next to your bathroom mirror, or anywhere else that you regularly pass by. Stop, take a look, and say to yourself "Oh yeah, that's me!".

Another approach is to take your vision board into the 21st century and make a vision movie. We have access to tons of images online and phones that can make beautiful movies with very little effort. (Although I do recommend having someone on hand who understands the technology - Yay to all of you who have a teenager in your life!). Use a search engine to find images that match a feeling you're working to manifest. You can literally search Google images for the word "serenity'" and come up with thousands of pictures that are representative of that sensation.

What I especially like about making a vision movie is that you can easily add music to it. This is where you can go back to our Power Playlist, take songs that evoke a higher energy frequency for yourself, and add images that fade in and out to produce a 3 - 5 minute movie. You can also use photos from your own library that make you smile. Set an alarm everyday to remind you to watch your movie. You'll be surprised how invigorating it can be! And whenever you wake up in a "Debbie downer" mood, taking a few minutes to watch your vision movie can be just the thing that immediately changes your viewpoint for the rest of the day.

You may want to consider making several vision movies: one for your career path, one for your relationship, one for your connection to the divine, etc. I've made short movies that were super specific, and also 6-minute ones that brought all aspects of my life together in one place. I suggest making one every six months or even once a year. Then when some of those things on your vision board or vision movie have manifested, it's time to make a new one!

5. Movement explorations to inspire you

My life has absolutely been inspired by movement. I've danced since I was 5 years old and I clearly remember that first ballet lesson. When I'm dancing, I experience a freedom unlike any other, and to this day it can uplift me with an expansiveness and a passion that nothing else has come close to. I used to think this was because I just love moving, but of course being the nerd that I am, I ended up researching the psychological effects of movement on the mind and emotions to discover what I already suspected: There is so much more going on that just some good ol' bum shaking!

I could write a whole other book on the importance of movement and how it stimulates your body, your brain, your hormones, and more so I won't go into the finer details here. You can check the Brahmaniyoga.com website for videos and the resources page for more in depth information on the benefits of movement. Also, a quick internet search will pull up thousands of articles to send you down the rabbit hole of movement research.

I do want to emphasise why *embodied* movement is meaningful and how it's an integral part of our personal transformation. Often we think of dance, yoga, sports, gymnastics, etc. in terms of what it looks like or achieving a desired outcome. But as I've discussed in the above section, we need to let go of constructed standards of right and wrong, move away from making pretty shapes or efficient movements, and embrace how we really feel in our bodies.

Simply stated, embodied yoga is having an awareness of how we feel internally when we are practicing. Our focus turns away from what we may look like and turns inward toward having a sensory experience. We take a journey through the body - listening, feeling, and noticing sensation and states of awareness that arise. Actually, any movement practice can be embodied, as long as we're not judging or predicting outcomes. So why is this relevant besides making us feel great? Because by applying an embodied practice, we change from using our analytical brain centre (the prefrontal cortex), instead firing up the sensory processors, like the thalamus and hippocampus. In this way, movement can become a meditation, which is not only therapeutic but also shifts our perspective on things.

To get you started I've created a 20 minute movement sequence that is playful and accessible for all. As I guide you to discover this sequence from an awareness of sensation, you'll get out of your mind and into your body. We'll finish with a brief meditation and also a journaling exercise.

Watch video number 6: "Embodied Movement Exploration"

6. Thinking outside the box

Some of the most creative moments happen when we think outside the box. We drop the "normal" view on an idea or concept and often find the perfect solution to a problem or get inspired to take a completely different direction.

"Boxes" are basically the accepted norms in any given community or industry or inherited through our families. If an idea falls outside of this realm, it's often considered to be too unconventional. But think about it: convention, the status quo, rules and regulations aren't there to inspire creativity or to allow people to really shine and excel. The norms are based on compliance to an ideal about behaviour, lifestyle, or even, ironically, to keep us safe.

Therefore, boxes often represent what is expected of us. And this is where so many of us get stuck. An expectation of something can kill our ability to bring new life or possibilities into our own identity. What does it look like to be a mother? A lawyer? A yoga teacher? When something has a label on it there are preconceived ideas and expectations associated with it.

It's like living according to that old saying: "if it ain't broke, don't fix it". I prefer what was written on the birthday card my dad got me this year, "Well behaved women never make history" (My dad gets me!).

Venturing to think outside the box is what has allowed our cultures and societies to grow and evolve. When someone in the past has had a seemingly outrageous idea, many will respond by saying it's impossible. But we know that's not true. Anything is possible with energy, belief and a healthy disregard for what others might think.

Today, flying in an airplane is a pretty standard way to get around when your destination is too far away to drive or take a train. But before the Wright Brothers came along and ignored everyone else, the idea that we could travel by air was considered preposterous. Extraordinary ideas have come from people who decided not to be confined by boxes or others' beliefs. And once a new invention or concept has been normalised, it allows other people to follow suit. On May 6, 1954 Roger Bannister broke the 4-minute mile at Oxford University. Up until that point, it was considered impossible to do. However since then, over 1400 runners worldwide have beat the 4-minute mark. So was it impossible? No, it just took someone to believe bigger, better, and beyond the box.

The lesson here is that when we're ready to evolve, learn something new, embark on a new journey or go in a new direction, we have to let go of the established norms in order to be open to all possibilities. Don't worry about what everyone else is doing, think bigger than that, smash the box and put it in the recycling bin!

"Instead of thinking outside the box, get rid of the box"

Deepak Chopra

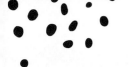

EXERCISES

The exercises below will help you to think outside the box, and therefore open up new alternatives. As the quote above attests, it's impossible to arrive at a different conclusion through an old mindset. Hopefully you'll discover that it's actually fairly simple to explore the possibilities, and that it's playful and kind of fun too.

Ask Children

It's logical to think *when in doubt ask an expert*, but if you really want to get beyond expectation and completely out of the box, try discussing your idea with someone between 3 - 7 years old. If you have kids you probably sense where I'm going with this. Children will often come up with some pretty hilarious responses to our 'adult' ideas and problems. But since at such a young age we haven't been completely conditioned by others' expectations, thinking outside the box is pretty normal at that stage. If you don't have children in this age group, ask your friends or relatives if you can have a conversation with their kids. Listen carefully and don't dismiss the craziest notions that children might present. Just start incorporating their responses into your thinking and see where this leads you.

The Idea Bounce

When we are ready to get in the arena with a big challenge, it's useful to bounce ideas back and forth with at least one other person. I recommend someone who you respect and is willing to see this as a fun game or like a school debate. This exercise is a variation on the *What if...?* journaling exercise from the Inner Critic section. You may even want to record the conversation and listen to it later to remember any ideas generated in the moment, and to probably have a good laugh too!

 Start off with your idea or project, stating it outloud to your friend (even if they already are aware of it).

 Your friend responds with a reason or two about why it's a bad idea.

 You will counter your friend's reasoning with a "What if...?" This "what if" should be all the reasons it could go perfectly well and end up even better than imagined. Don't hold back.

 Your friend then challenges that as well and they can also get outrageous. You carry on going back and forth, having fun pushing each other until you're exhausted and hopefully laughing a lot.

Example:

Me: What if I were to start a yoga studio in India even though I have no business experience there, not completely sure what it entails, and I'll be leaving behind a credible following of students in the UK?

My Friend: It's a bad idea because Indians won't take your classes, so who are you going to teach?

Me: What if my students were to come over from Europe since many Europeans travel to India to go on holiday and learn yoga?

My Friend: OK, but you still must be crazy because you don't speak the language and you have no idea about running a business.

Me: What if I learned everything I could before setting it up, and then find some helpful people once I arrive? I wouldn't be the first Westerner to set up a business in India.

My Friend: It's so risky. What if it fails?

Me: What if it succeeds?

This tool is meant to keep bouncing different ideas around while exploring the initial challenge. It's not about agreeing with your friend. It's about you each keeping your own sides to flesh out all the possibilities in both trains of thought. We often can be sucked into someone's list of reasons not to do something because it sounds logical at first. But remember, there will also be a long list of great reasons why you absolutely should do your thing.

You might have guessed that the example above is my own personal experience. It didn't really dawn on me how outrageous the idea was at the time. I'm a white western woman who decides to move to India, set up a big yoga centre, and teach there. Sounds crazy right? Well, luckily I stuck with my gut instinct because I didn't really get a solid reason NOT to do it when I threw the idea around with my friends. This is how Brahmani Yoga was born, and it became one of the most successful yoga centres in Goa from 2005 to 2012. It wasn't easy, but it was rewarding and allowed me to grow as a teacher and as a business owner. It also made me realise that I was capable of much more than I had previously thought. Even more so, the European yoga teachers who came to Brahmani started inviting me to teach at their studios all over Europe. This was how I became an international traveling yoga teacher. It would have never happened if I had listened to someone else's reasons not to follow my dream.

Ask The Plumber

OK I know this sounds a little silly, but what I mean here is talk to someone who works in a completely different industry than you. We often throw around our ideas and ambitions with friends and colleagues who know the ins and outs of what we do. Of course there's nothing wrong with this, and it's always beneficial to seek advice from someone with a lot of experience in your field. However, when we want to shift perspective it can be super useful to talk to someone who would have a completely different outlook on the matter. You want to create your own interior design company after working for another firm? Talk to someone who sells cars. Thinking of becoming a real estate agent? Talk to someone who does public speaking events. Get the gist? Someone who isn't familiar with your chosen subject will usually ask questions and give suggestions that might not occur to you simply because they are "outside of your box", per se.

I've experienced for myself how useful this can be. I have a student who is a retired investment broker and has run 3 different companies. When I talk to him about a project I'm working on, he always points out how to make the ideas bigger, how to reach more people, or how essential it is that I weave science into my work but to make it accessible so that everyone can easily understand it. He really pushes me to expand my thinking into other realms, and it's reaffirming that I'm on the right track to reach yoga teachers and the general public - which is one of my goals!

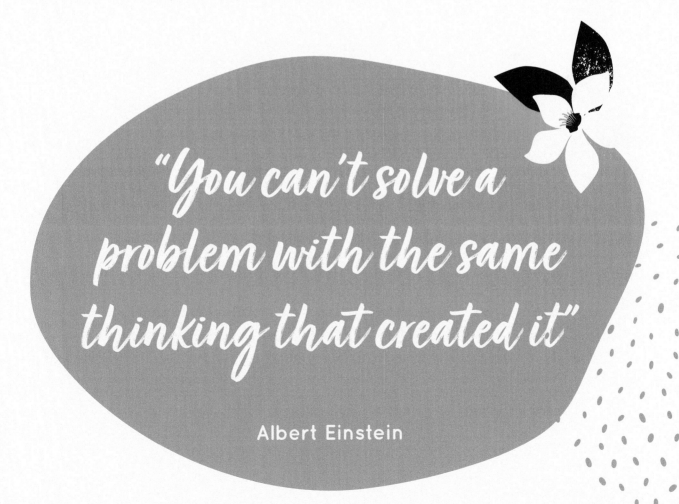

"You can't solve a problem with the same thinking that created it"

Albert Einstein

7. Pranayama - Breath work to focus our energy

Pranayama (yogic breathing exercises) techniques are excellent for clearing the mind and focusing energy. Previously kept as the secret tradition of master yogis, we now understand the connection between the nervous system and the breath, and how it can be used to calm and to heal. Some of the more common breathing techniques are used in Navy Seal training, prison projects, and in some classrooms to help relieve anxiety and stress.

In this video I will take you through a technique where we extend the exhale a little longer than the inhale. This is a practice in yoga known as Vi-Sama Vritti and has been touted as being extremely beneficial. But even recent research by non-yoga practitioners shows that the science behind extending the exhale longer than the inhale is worth investigation.

I highly recommend James Nestor's book *Breath - The New Science of a Lost Art* (see Resources). He describes research into the extension of the exhales and how this triggers the parasympathetic nervous system (your rest and digest mode) and has a calming effect on the entire body. Any techniques we can engage in that counter balance stress in our lives is going to be useful.

Due to the relaxation you'll feel once you've completed this exercise, it will be a perfect time for you to engage with one of your creative endeavours. You'll have a clearer mind and be in a head space to see more possibilities.

Follow along with the video and see how you feel afterward. This is a practice you can do everyday for 10 minutes or even once a week.

Watch video number 7: "Pranayama - Extending exhales"

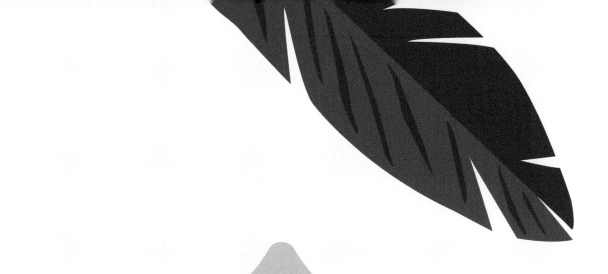

"Something is impossible only until one person has done it. From that point on it becomes possible for anyone to do it. Don't underestimate yourself. Maybe that one person is you."

Julie Martin

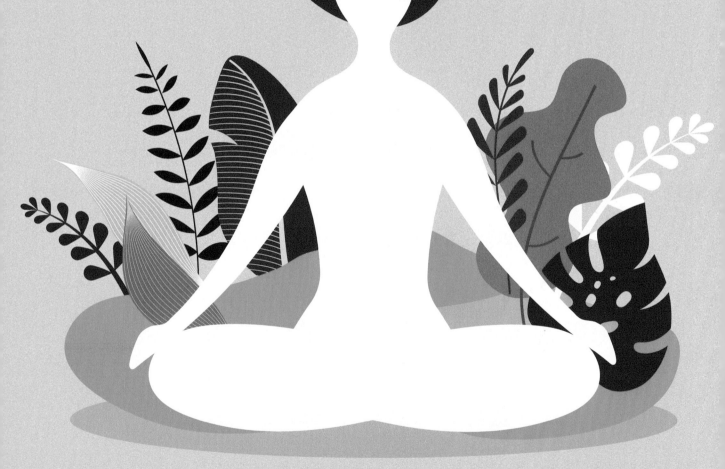

"*Everything is interesting, you just have to look closer.*"

Leonard Cohen

3. Implementing and maintaining growth

If you've made it this far, hopefully you've been exploring a lot of the exercises from the previous sections discovering what works for you and what you might leave for later. It's kind of like being left alone in a shoe store, right? You've been trying on different options for size, comfort, and some just for the fun of it. Perfect!

So now the big question is: "How do I use all these great tools and techniques and maintain the momentum to continue to focus on my inner growth and expansion?"

Does this scenario sound familiar: You've been on a roll journaling, meditating, doing movement practices and some of the other exercises in this workbook, then something changes in your environment that pulls your attention and your energy, so you take a temporary break from all of this. Next thing you know, days, weeks, and months have gone by and this workbook has gotten buried on a shelf somewhere gathering dust.

No, I don't have a crystal ball and I'm definitely not rooting against you. I just know how tricky the mind can be as it tries to distract us.

Remember our limbic system loves efficiency. And transformation takes time, conscientious effort, and mindful use of energy - all of which are seemingly inefficient to your limbic system. It's going to pipe up and ask, cajole, and maybe even scream at you to just go back to your old belief systems and the limiting ways of perceiving yourself and your potential. Doing so will in fact feel familiar, easier, and therefore, comforting. Then maybe your eye alights upon this workbook again, the old belief systems kick in, and your mind is off on a detrimental tangent of, "I'm such a loser-slacker-unworthy person who doesn't deserve transformation in my life".

OK, so how to get back on track? Or, for those of you moving right along, how do you maintain your momentum? I don't like to use the word "discipline" because it tends to evoke negative connotations. It brings us into a "I should" dialogue, and I like to live by the mantra "don't should all over yourself'. Certainly it's important to do these exercises regularly, but it's not about discipline at all. It's about making a commitment to yourself. It's about asking yourself, "How do I show up for myself and who I want to be TODAY?". Keep returning to your practices and tools and know that each challenge - each moment you may want to stop and go back to sitting on the sofa to binge watch TV - is actually a moment to grow. A moment to learn from. An opportunity to say to your former self "That's not who I am anymore, but thanks for trying".

This section is all about staying committed to your transformation, understanding the pitfalls you may encounter, and how to shift your perception to stay on track constructively and lovingly. Essentially, you'll learn how to cultivate a life that is a journey instead of a series of goals to be met. You might meet your goals, but the importance of a life well lived is that you are truly living it from your heart and body.

1. Befriending and embracing the unknown

One of the biggest challenges we often face is not knowing what's coming next. It's the source of many peoples' fears. We think we are secure and stable as long we have a plan and everything is going according to that plan. But we all know that circumstances change - we lose jobs, we have a break-up from a relationship, someone else changes their mind about a project we were working on together. The truth is there's no such thing as security: It's a concept and that's about it.

It's so easy to be thrown off course when the unexpected happens, and yet my reminder to others is always that this is where the practice begins. That is the truth. When we're doing great and everything is falling into place it's easy, we're motivated, we're seeing results, we're in tune with ourselves. The hardest moments are when we've had the rug pulled from under our feet and nothing seems to be working.

So how do we embrace the unknown? Well, start with the understanding that we are always living in the unknown and security is an illusion. We may have insurance, a roof over our head, a great job and family, but if the Covid-19 pandemic taught us anything it's that everything can become uncertain overnight. However, when we can recognize with our entire being - mind, body, and soul - that we are equipped with the tools, power, wisdom, and support to get through whatever may come our way, then we can trust. From there, the creative empowerment tools help us adapt or change things that might show us possibilities we never imagined.

Resistance vs Yielding

My first recommendation is to let go of resistance and yield to situations you can't control. In movement, yielding to the body allows us to find ease in our strength without brute force. This is a lesson for how to approach life in general. In a moment of uncertainty, we may want to dig in our heels and think, "No, no, no, no this has to go back to the way I planned it". However, not only is this reaction futile in most situations, it also makes our cortisol levels rise as we move into stress mode. For those who work in an environment where there are a lot of moving parts that don't always synchronise, this resistance and subsequent cortisol spike can be a weekly or even daily experience.

We can change how we view these types of situations. When that unexpected glitch happens what if the first thing we say to ourselves is "This is interesting, I didn't know that was going to happen"? Remember in the last section when we wrote about things that initially seemed bad and then became turning points that led us into a different direction, often for the better? It is possible to always be in that investigative mode. Instead of seeing the unknown as scary or disastrous, we can label it as "interesting" and drop the expectations.

Surviving vs Thriving

Once we have a curious outlook on our lives, then we can shift from the feeling of fear - which is a survival technique - to actual thriving. The survival of any species is not about strength; it's about adaptability. We're still on this planet because individuals and societies were able to adapt and change, and see this process in a positive light. Trying new things, experimenting, thinking outside the box, and engaging in playtime can help us see the possibilities in everything. Where someone might only observe an obstacle, we can find creativity.

I have a friend who is a interior designer. You walk into his house and it's amazing. Everything is beautiful and at first sight you'd think he spent hundreds of thousands on decor. But he'll talk you through almost every piece in his house, and you'll find that most of it was old and discarded stuff that he turned into magnificent furniture, curtains, mirrors, kitchen cabinets, etc. He takes the concept of 'One man's trash is another man's treasure' into the realm of a 5 star hotel!

Another example, when Covid-19 first locked us all up in our homes some businesses went straight into thriving mode. Lucky for the world we already had the technology. Online meetings, classes, courses, even doctors appointments became the norm. Those professionals or businesses that didn't take so kindly to being online, to figuring out which camera to use, or how to sort out their sound have been left in deeper uncertainty.

I mentor a lot of yoga teachers and I found that while everyone was thrown into initial fear mode, those who decided to bite the bullet and learn new IT skills have been able to continue to do what they love, with some of them even thriving more than before. This was certainly the case for me, too, as my steady income was based on traveling to Europe and other places to teach workshops and trainings. My first few weeks online we're frustrating and annoying as I had to learn a lot in a short amount of time. Who knew that in less than one month I'd have to figure out how to light my room, get music to continue to play when I was speaking on camera, while ensuring everyone could see what I was doing? But I knew I had to do it in order to continue to reach my students. The initial difficulties have given me more confidence, and now I find myself saying "You've got this Julie. You'll figure it out" when something technical doesn't work or I'm faced with a new platform to learn.

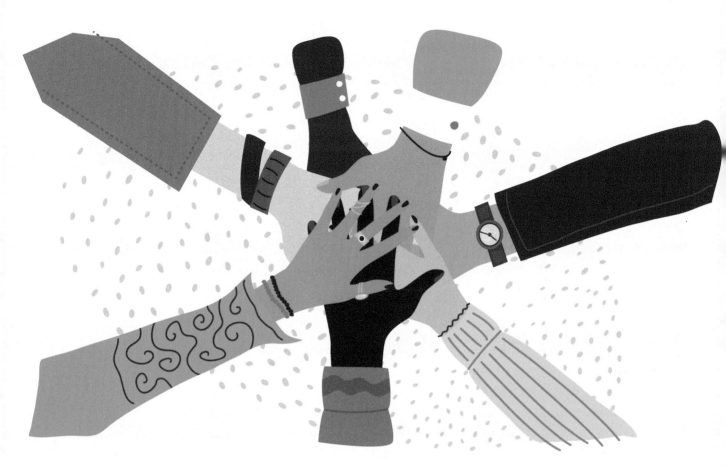

2. Community = common + unity

Our ability to find our grounding and to thrive is absolutely dependent on who is around to support us. You may have noticed that many of the exercises in this book involve working with a friend or a group of friends. Some of the basic aspects of community are that we receive encouragement, connection, and assistance. And we can have different communities for different areas of our lives. Most of us have a trusted group of friends as our most important community being that they know us more intimately than others. Another community can be found in our field of work or career area. Then there's our religious/spiritual community, our playtime community, workout community, creative community, etc. Alcoholics Anonymous and AlAnon (for the friends and family of alcoholics) have built their entire structure on the importance of community support. Community lets us know that we're not alone, that others have had similar experiences and can serve as a sounding board, a helping hand, and an understanding heart.

An article in *National Alliance on Mental Illness* titled "The Importance of Community and Mental Health", Stephanie Gilbert writes: "Community is not just an entity or a group of people, it's a feeling. It's feeling connected to others, feeling accepted for who you are and feeling supported"[5].

Additional research into mental health, longevity, and general wellbeing also emphasises the value of community. In fact, while we may perceive loners as being mysterious, windswept, and interesting, the studies show that they're the most likely to suffer from depression and long-term anxiety.

Having a solid sense of belonging is another main aspect of community. Through her research, Brené Brown describes that there is a vast difference between fitting in and belonging. In her book *The Gifts of Imperfection* she states, "Fitting in is about assessing a situation and becoming who you need to be to be accepted. Belonging, on the other hand, doesn't require us to change who we are; it requires us to be who we are"[6].

We tend to know early on where we belong. Often families and our early friendships offer us this sanctuary. For me, while I really enjoyed dance from an early age, I didn't necessarily belong to the community of dancers where I was taking classes from since they were all skinny pale girls who looked like they stepped right out of *The Nutcracker*. But when I started up at a different studio with a teacher who I had heard wonderful things about, I could feel myself relax and just let go by the end of the first class. I was being taught through encouragement instead of being held to the standard of a classical ballerina (which clearly I was not!). I felt like she believed in me and in every other student there. Needless to say, that woman became a lifelong mentor, and it was there that I found my best friend forever, who still makes me feel like I belong wherever I go.

Community also gives us a sense of purpose. Communities usually form through common goals and a sense of purposeful work. For example: being in a choir that gives an annual concert where members will support each other through the rehearsal process and the pre-show nerves, or being a part of a church or a charity organisation that creates events for holidays or other special occasions. Situations like these help us build trust in teamwork, which is really valuable for recovering perfectionists and those who put pressure on themselves to 'do it all'.

Whenever we waiver or doubt ourselves or our endeavours, community plays that vital role to keep us going forward. A strong, supportive community can keep us on track, provide accountability without judgement, and be a safe place to just be ourselves.

EXERCISE

Identify the different communities in your life. Mentally evaluate each one to see how it makes you feel and determine if you're gaining a true sense of belonging as opposed to just fitting in. Some of you may feel totally supported in every way by your friends and/or family, but it's also essential to have community outside of those realms. If you are a yoga or movement teacher have regular check-ins with other trusted teachers. If you feel isolated in what you do, seek out other people involved in similar endeavors such as your hobbies, religion, or career field (especially for those of you who are self-employed and/or working from home, which can often be a lonely place). Anything from a book club to a mental health support group can be that network that helps to provide grounding, purpose, and belonging.

On the left side of your Gratitude Journal make sure that you write how grateful you feel for the communities that support you. If you begin to notice that one or more of the groups that you are involved with are no longer serving a purpose it may be time to move on. You'll know when you write in your journal about it. It just won't *feel* right.

3. Setting Boundaries

If I could go back in time and have a class on setting boundaries when I was in my formative years, it would have been a life-changer. I suspect I'm not alone in this. Whether you recognise it or not, we've all been brought up in an environment that teaches us to please others in order to feel validation. First and foremost, our parents' approval motivated us to follow household rules and regulations. For those who have stable and emotionally-balanced parents, then following household rules develops into a basic understanding of respect. However, in households where the rules are thinly veiled manifestations of our parents' fears meant to provide "safety" through control, the idea of respect becomes rooted in fearing a lack of approval.

When we get to school the approval ante is upped a notch or two. First, we want to do well to please both our parents and our teachers. If we're not performing well, we get reprimanded which often leads to shame (because it's typically delivered publicly and disparagingly). Then there's wanting to be liked in order to build and maintain friendships (See above about Community). Of course we desperately want to belong, which can mean pushing ourselves to exhaustion to overperform, or being the class clown and getting in trouble, or even underperforming to gain approval from our circle of peers.

Many of us never outgrow these feelings from our childhoods. So it's no surprise that one of the things I notice in adults across the board, regardless of their vocation or what stage of life they're in, is that they have an extremely hard time setting healthy boundaries. In fact, they often don't set any boundaries at all or go to the extreme of constructing a full suit of boundary armour. This exists for two main reasons: 1) Fear of not being accepted, liked, or being validated, and 2) fear of losing control.

Because we crave approval (often subconsciously) setting boundaries is tricky, especially with friends, colleagues you've known a long time, and definitely with new bosses and employers. Ever set up a business venture with good friends thinking it would be fun? Well, you've probably felt the sting of assuming everyone would be on the same page regarding behaviour and protocols. Then we're afraid to say something for fear of losing our friends. However, what often happens is that the friendships do fall apart, or the business does, or both. This is why setting boundaries from the onset is vital. Yes, we may be friends but let's make sure we all know what's expected of each other throughout the process of reaching common goals.

The same goes for family members. Whether it's about weighing in on your relationship status, your child-rearing skills (a tough one I know many people have a hard time with), or quitting your job to focus on something you truly love, families that lack healthy boundaries can often decide it's their place to take over where you "clearly don't have the skills or experience" or they simply think you've gone crazy. As adults we definitely need to set healthy boundaries with our parents. They tend to still look at us as if we're 5 years old and need them for everything (those of you with grown children experience the other end of this). Remember that no one is in charge of your life but you. Advice is one thing, but pressure to do what they think is best is never going to result in a balanced relationship or your own growth.

It's in dealing with the workplace where I see the greatest need for setting boundaries. Employer/employee, client/provider, teacher/(adult) student are all relationships that can go pretty haywire without clear boundaries. In a world where many of us are self-employed or have jobs where we work at least part-time from home, the boundaries often get blurred. We can feel the need to be available 24/7 in order to please clients or employers, and yet this is what gets us out of balance and stressed. The knock-on effect is that our other relationships suffer for it as well.

If we're on the road to transformation then this area is like a large roundabout that we need to get to the other side of. And yes, we will probably circle back around a few times as we learn. What it boils down to is good communication. But because the conversations we need to have are usually with people we deeply love or respect or are signing our paycheck, or both, we will feel vulnerable. The biggest worries? We won't be liked anymore. We'll lose friends. We'll get in trouble from someone "higher up", we'll lose clients, etc. And yet, when we encounter people who set clear boundaries we usually respect them more and can build trust with them because we know where they stand. This is what we want to bear in mind as we move into our strength.

Since it all boils down to communication, it's vital to be as clear as possible about what you want, or expect from the other(s) involved. Understand that saying *No* or disagreeing doesn't mean a friendship or work relationship has to end. Also in some circumstances, setting boundaries involves negotiation, which means being heard and being open to hearing what the other is saying. Conversely, if you feel your needs are being dismissed or you're being told "you're too selfish", then it might be time to cut the ties with that relationship/job/client. Remember, you're not responsible for how the other person feels about your needs. Implementing growth is about moving beyond being a people-pleaser and setting healthy parameters to move forward. The following exercises will help you to evaluate your boundaries to ensure they are working for you and to establish new ones, if needed.

EXERCISES

Professional Boundaries
If you are really passionate about what you do, it can be really problematic to set boundaries. So often we dismiss the work overload or the need to be constantly accessible because we 'love' our jobs. However, you can be headed towards burnout no differently than someone who doesn't really like what they do; it just might take a little longer.

If you're self-employed you can set boundaries using some simple measures. Ensure that your website and contract state clear working hours. This way if you don't answer that email or text at 1:00 am, your clients will learn that you respond when you have specified you're available. If you have a private client who loves to talk with you after their session is over and doesn't seem to have an 'off' button, that needs to be nipped in the bud. Clients will often turn to you as a sounding board or psychotherapist, which becomes an energy drain if that's not part of your job. Tell them that while you'd love to hear what they have to say, you have another client in 10 minutes (this doesn't have to be true). It reminds them that your availability is limited to their session and your scheduled work hours.

Furthermore, it can be anxiety inducing to set fees or ask for a pay raise, and here is where you want to check in with what you genuinely feel you are worth. What is your level of experience? What kind of commitment are you making? Look back at your Life Closet, Gratitude Journal, and Shine List to make sure you are focusing on earning what you deserve. Yes, it's super scary at first to be straightforward about what you will deliver and what you expect to be paid, but it's also incredibly empowering once you get on the other side of it!

Lastly, there's working as part of a team. Do all team members precisely understand what is expected of them and what they can expect from the team leader? Frank conversations about boundaries (i.e. who does what) and expectations (timelines, thoroughness, communication among the team, etc.) can save hours of energy normally wasted on assumptions.

Family and Friend Boundaries

One of the hardest areas to set boundaries is with those we love and who love us. Nevertheless, sometimes a family member or friend constantly crosses the line, or they have an idea of who they think you should be and continue to get annoyed when you don't meet their expectations. These conversations need to be handled with care and sensitivity, but most importantly, they need to be handled. It's so easy to bury these conversations under the rug, yet our growth requires us to let others know how we feel.

Setting boundaries with family means having all involved parties sit down together for a discussion. You open by sharing how you are affected by the others' comments or expectations, however, in order to set healthy boundaries all parties need to be heard. Everyone gets to participate in the conversation, and if any disagreements arise then negotiate toward a solution that all are comfortable with. Keep in mind that with family it will never be black and white, and some people may initially get offended. Start with a caring yet strong opener ike "I love you and value our relationship but I need to express something that is bothering me and I feel we need to establish some clear boundaries". You might even be surprised that the other party/parties had no idea they were crossing the line or making you feel unhappy and they sincerely apologise, allowing everyone involved to learn and grow from the experience.

Setting boundaries with friends also presents its challenges. Do any of these scenarios sound familiar: someone's always asking for favours but never returns them? Friends who cancel at the last minute all the time? Or someone who expects you to pick up the phone no matter what time and gets miffed when you don't? If these are friends who we love and trust despite their shortcomings (and we all have them), then setting boundaries will only strengthen the relationship.

I personally have a quirk where if I'm out with friends and I'm ready to go home, I often just get up, grab my bag, wave, and leave. I hate doing the 20 minute goodbye dialogue "Well, I better be going. It was great seeing you, I had fun. Yes, we should do it again soon. Steve? Yeah, I remember him. He's running a marathon next Sunday? Everyone's going?" - at this point I'm dying. While my friends know this about me, I still remind them before going out together. And when I meet new friends, I tell them in advance about my quirk so there are no surprises. They might not even see me leave, but I'll always call the next day and let them know that I enjoyed myself and look forward to the next time.

Self Boundaries

We often forget to set our own self boundaries. If we're the most important person in our lives (and we are), then we need to look after Number One. Setting your own personal boundaries is about making sure you have the time and energy for everything you want to do. If you promised yourself a holiday but let your dedication to work override it, you need to put your foot down. If you want more time in your day for personal stuff but find you've scheduled many social events in addition to work and home chores, that's you mishandling your own timing.

I am the queen of overscheduling myself, and I'm still learning to say *No*. I can open my calendar on a Monday morning and look at all the private clients, mentees, and classes I've scheduled, the lunch I promised to do with the neighbour, plus I told someone I'd help feed their baby sheep, and I need to write up documents for a teacher training. I'll put my head in my hands and think, "Who scheduled all of this in one day?". The resounding answer from above is, "You, sister! YOU did this. In fact, you have us in stitches most weeks!". Yes, it's all my own doing. But that also means it's my own undoing as well. I have to pause before responding to requests - professional and personal - because my initial reaction is usually "Sure!". What I really need to say and do is, "Let me check my schedule and I'll get back to you on that". And if it's simply too much to do in a day and I'm not leaving myself any time for myself, then a compassionate *No* is the only acceptable response.

4. Being in service to others

We are never more in a place of receiving as when we are in service to others. That may sound contradictory, but when we take the time and energy to help others we're telling the Universe that we have the time, energy and even the funds to be in this moment for the greater good. Why is this so powerful? When we turn our attention away from our own dilemmas and focus on others' wellbeing we realise how good we have it ourselves, and that we have the capacity to help someone else experience some of it. We are being useful, not because we want to be liked or validated, but simply for the sake of showing up for others, and that can be healing for both parties.

Being in service is referred to as Seva in the yoga world. Usually translated as 'selfless service', the literal meaning of Seva is 'together with', which I love because it also suggests an aspect of unity.

Selfless service can take a variety of forms. While the first thing that may pop into your head is working for a charity or volunteering for a nonprofit organisation, there are a multitude of ways we can show up for others without expecting anything in return. Here are a just a few suggestions:

Offer your professional services for free
Since I teach yoga, train yoga teachers, and mentor people, I have a lot of opportunities to be there for others when they can't afford to attend events or invest in training. Being self-employed means that I can easily omit my fees when I discover that someone needs some help. I remember many years ago shifting my perspective away from being a "successful yoga teacher" who has a large following, to ensuring that people walked away inspired, empowered, and in control of their own transformation. When it became obvious that this was the goal for me as a teacher, it was also clear that it couldn't be limited to only those who could afford it.

Help out a friend or neighbour
It can sound so simple but often just giving our time to someone who needs a helping hand or an ear to listen to their stories, makes a huge impact on them. While we live in a time where we don't really know our neighbours, I feel it's integral to have connection with those people living around us. Not only for the sake of community, but also to be aware of eldery or infirm neighbours who might need some assistance now and again, especially if they're living alone.

Get involved as a Big Brother or Big Sister
Children who grow up in single-parent families where that parent is overworked are at higher risk for drug use, dropping out of school, and

having low self-esteem. These programs are designed to match a child from an underprivileged environment with an adult mentor who can help them with their school work, take them out for cultural experiences, and just hang out together. The impact on the kids and their parents is extraordinary and has a lasting effect. In the United States the organisation can be found at https://www.bbbs.org. Similar organisations exist throughout the world.

Mentor a newcomer in your field

I'm pretty sure that if you take a look back on your life, you can name a person or two who took you under their wing and helped you get to where you are now. By sharing your time, experience, and expertise to nurture the next generation's talent, you can keep this flow of energy moving forward while reminding yourself of your own humble beginning and how having a mentor helped smooth the road ahead for you.

Volunteer at an animal shelter or foster a pet

Working with animals can be so rewarding. There are many stories about people who rescued animals to discover that the animal actually saved them. Of course there is the danger (certainly in my case) of adopting as many cats and dogs as your house can hold. Still, those pets will always be grateful.

Random acts of kindness go a long way

I love the idea of paying it forward and random acts of kindness. If we don't have a lot of time to dedicate to a bigger project to be of service, we can do small things everyday to lift others' spirits. Buy a coffee for the stranger behind you in line. Hold the door open for a parent pushing a pram/stroller. Let someone go ahead of you when you can sense that they're in a hurry. You can make a big difference in someone's day just by doing some small thing that makes their day easier.

These are just a few ideas on how to be in service with the understanding that the ways in which we can give our time, energy, and money are limitless. The only guideline here is that it is not about our own gain, it's about serving others and ultimately society at large as we restore faith in humanity.

5. The Gift Box

The Gift Box is a simple and yet very rewarding tool. The name pretty much says it all. You'll create a Gift Box for yourself, from yourself, and it will be filled with inspirational moments you've had.

The instructions are easy: Find a nice box that is small enough to keep by your bed. It should be a box that looks like it holds something special (because it will!), so that you feel delighted when you see it.

Next: Notice when you do something you're proud of. It may be making a positive choice during your day, the results of a project/job/course you've been working on, or even catching yourself employing a new tool to break the cycle of your old belief system. You might find yourself feeling confident in a moment that would normally make you anxious, graciously accepting a compliment, receiving an unsolicited hug from a loved one with a fully open heart, or simply sharing a laugh with some close friends. Anything that you are truly grateful for when you think back on it at the end of the day. Write down these things on small pieces of paper whenever you remember. Fold them up and put them in your Gift Box. These are your gifts. Collect as many of these 'wins' as you like and fill that box to the maximum. The act itself of noticing and taking the time to acknowledge your 'gift' on paper will bring higher vibrations into your being.

Then on days when you're not feeling 100% and like nothing is really working for you, reach into your Gift Box and read some of your accomplishments and happy moments. Do this before going to bed so that the last thing that crosses your mind before you go to sleep is a really positive memory. Remind yourself that if you've done well before, you'll do well again. Today may have just been a slow day for you and that's OK.

And of course, you can read a note from your Gift Box any time if you feel you need some inspiration. If you have children this is also a great practice for them.

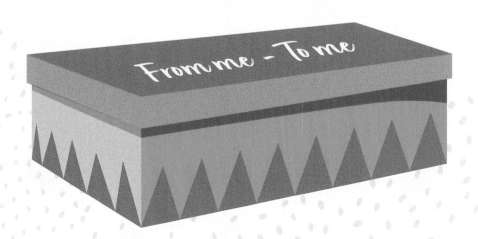

6. Journaling our progress - *'I believe in myself'*

We are going to do this journaling exercise together via the video below. First, we'll do some movement to get out of our 'thinking' minds and relax the nervous system. Then we'll pick up our journals and I'll give you a task of writing without any conscious thinking. Sounds a bit strange, I know, but trust me. The video will guide you through and you'll find the results pretty surprising.

Watch video number 8: "Journaling Exercise"

7. Pranayama - Tibetan purification

This is one of my favourite breathing exercises. It's a variation on alternate nostril breathing and it will bring the mind and the body into balance with ease. You don't have to have deep lung capacity and you won't be holding your breath (I know some people find that really challenging). This exercise includes what we call a mudra as we'll use the movement of the hand to reflect the movement of the breath. Most people find it beautiful to do and love coming back to it again and again. I'll guide you through the whole process as we practice together with the video.

Watch video number 9: "Pranayama - Tibetan Purification"

8. Heart centre meditation

This meditation is about coming home to ourselves. Our connection with compassion - whether it's for someone else or ourselves - is truly vital for our overall well being. Not only can we find peace and calm when we focus on the energy of the heart centre, it automatically lowers our cortisol levels and heart rate, thus boosting the immune system. The meditation is loosely based on the Bhuddist Metta meditation technique, as we direct our love and compassion toward other people and ourselves. I'll take you through the whole sequence in the video so get comfortable when you're ready to start.

Watch video number 10: "Heart Centre Meditation"

Find a comfortable place to sit and take a moment to notice how your body feels in this position. Do a body scan from bottom to top and sense where there may be tension and ask your body to release it. Don't judge it if you have a difficult time releasing this tension. Take a moment to swallow to relax your jaw and throat. Soften your eyebrows and forehead.

- Begin to notice your breath as it is for a few minutes, there's no need to change it. Then take your awareness to your heart centre (in the centre of your chest not the anatomical heart which is slightly to the left). You might sense a sensation there. It can be anything: the rhythm of your breath, the beating of your heart, or just how the energy feels in that part of your body. You can't get this wrong, whatever you're sensing is correct.

- Now think of someone who you really love and who loves you. Hold them in your heart and see if the energy rises. What feelings do you get when you think of them? You might even find yourself smiling. Hold onto this feeling for 5 minutes or more. You can even go through a few people who you really love, it doesn't have to be just one.

- The next step is to think of someone who you know needs some help and compassion. It can be a friend in need or a person you are just familiar with but you know their story. Hold them in your heart centre with the same energy that you held the previous person/s for 3-5 minutes.

- Now we move on to a person who truly challenges you. Someone that you have friction with or outright makes you angry. (Yes, this is the most difficult part of the practice.) Hold them in your heart centre. You've already cultivated the energy of love and compassion so visualise yourself surrounding this person with that same energy. Drop the internal dialogue that you have with them. Take about 3-5 minutes for this section.

- Finally, place yourself in your own heart centre and give yourself the same love and compassionate energy that you have held for everyone else. Let it radiate to all of your cells. See them light up from within. Feel all of your organs shining light, your skin glowing with light, and you being surrounded by loving light. Rest there for 3-5 minutes as well.

- As we finish, let go of that imagery and bring yourself back to the present moment. Notice your sit bones on the floor or chair once again. Deepen your breath for a few rounds and then slowly blink your eyes open.

Doing this meditation regularly will truly bring you into a compassionate relationship with yourself and others around you. You'll even notice that the people who challenge you, will start to behave differently once they've been brought into the meditation.

9. You Have Permission to Do Nothing

This may sound a bit crazy and somewhat contradictory to the rest of the book, but in fact it's a vital part of our progress. Because we've created a society that encourages us to do more and be more productive we can bring that mindset into our journey of transformation, which isn't really helpful. It's a mindset we need to examine if it's our default.

There will be days, weeks, months or even more where you will feel lost, confused, ready to crawl back under the covers and stay forever. I'm here to tell you that's okay and it's totally normal. Recognise and embrace the simple truth - we need breaks. We need to put things on hold. It's actually part of maintaining momentum in our process. Less is more because we give ourselves breathing space to step back and observe. It also allows our nervous system to recalibrate.

When we stop, whether that is the entire process or just one aspect, we give our brains and bodies time to just rest in the information that we have learned and experienced so far. Taking time to do nothing becomes really powerful when it's intentional. Giving yourself a set amount of time 'off' will bring a new perspective and awareness when you get back to the work. I'll illustrate with an example.

As a mentor to yoga teachers I am constantly coming across 'teachers burnout'. This can be anything from just not feeling like they fit into the yoga world or lacking inspiration and wanting to give it all up. It happens to all of us at some point when you are doing something that you love and therefore have a deeply personal connection to it. So I prescribe intentional 'do nothing' time. I had one mentee who was deeply uninspired with her teaching and practice. So I told her to do absolutely no yoga whatsoever for a whole month. No teaching, no practice, no creating sequences, nothing. She was allowed to do other forms of movement and could teach her mindfulness classes, just not the asana which she was getting frustrated with. At the end of the month, when she returned to her practice it was with a sense of newness. A new beginning and she was inspired to get back into it because she was able to experience the practice with a fresh outlook.

The key to this non-action phase is that you have permission. I'm telling you right now – "Go for it!". But make a commitment to that time off, don't dabble when you're tempted. If you decide it's a week or a month off then stick to it. If we continue to dabble and listen to the voice that says maybe I should, then we're back to square one, usually feeling guilty. Enjoy your time off, like any vacation or holiday and return rested, renewed and hopefully re-inspired.

Watch video number 11: "Bonus Video- Anytime Daily Reset"

This is where the practice begins

Congratulations on getting this far. Every time I read back through the book I think, "Wow, that's a lot!". And it is. But this is a journey and there are no rules and regulations about how quickly you need to get through all the exercises, and of course there is no right outcome. There is only your individual experience of it. Some of the exercises might really speak to you and so you repeat them often and others might warrant a 'Meh'. Personal growth is such an individual thing that we can't really pinpoint the perfect combination of things to get us through. It will always be an investigation, and if that's your biggest take-away from this workbook, then it's already a lot.

My hope is that you now have this amazing tool box to guide you, keep you moving forward, and keep you staying grounded at the same time. If we can find more ease in our own lives, we project that ease to those around us too. We can find a greater harmony. But don't get me wrong, I definitely know that there will be days, weeks, and months where everything seems like it's all an uphill climb. If we can take those moments and remind ourselves that this is part of the growth, and a vital part of it, we'll come out of it on the other side having learned something about ourselves.

To close, I just want to share my gratitude for you, with you. It has always been an honour for me to help others, to guide those who need a hand, and to celebrate with you when you find those precious moments of triumph however large or small. As you continue your journey I'm there with you in spirit, cheering you on, and shouting, **You've got this!**

Thank you

References:

1. John Kim (Containers analogy for recognising areas of your life that you want to examine) - From the JRNI Coaching Course

2. Anne Pyburn Craig - *Creative Development in Early Childhood* (https://classroom.synonym.com/creative-developmentearlchildhood-6403534.html)

3. Laura D. Newpoff - *American Nurse - Creative wellness: A missing link in boosting well-being* (https://www.myamericannurse.com/creativewellness-boosting-wellbeing)

4. Hara Estroff Marano - *Psychology today - The Power of Play* (https://www.psychologytoday.com/us/articles/199907/the-power-play)

5. Stephanie Gilvert - *The Importance of Community and Mental Health* (https://nami.org/Blogs/NAMI-Blog/November-2019/The-Importance-of-Community-and-Mental-Health)

6. Brené Brown - *The Gifts of Imperfection*

Resources:

THE FOUR PILLARS OF TRANSFORMATION

Pema Chodron - *Start where you are*

Brené Brown - *Daring Greatly: How the Courage to Be Vulnerable Transforms the Way We Live*, and her Ted Talk *The Power of Vulnerability*

Dr. Joe Dispenza - *Breaking the Habit of being yourself* and *Becoming Supernatural*

Amy Cuddy - *Presence*, and her Ted Talk *Your body language may shape who you are*

Louise Hay - *You can Heal Your Life*

Alli Hoff Kosik - *Why Dancing is Good for your Brain* (https://www.theladders.com/career-advice/heres-why-dancing-is-good-foryour-brain)

CREATIVE EMPOWERMENT

Julia Cameron - *The Artist's Way*

Betty Edwards - *Drawing on the Right Side of the Brain*

Stuart Brown - Ted Talk *Play is more than just Fun*

Jennifer Wallace - Washington Post - *Why it's Good for Grown-ups to go Play* (https://www.washingtonpost.com/national/health-science/why-its-good-for-grown-ups-to-go-play/2017/05/19/99810292-fd1f-11e6-8ebe-6e0dbe4f2bca_story.html)

James Nestor - *Breath: The New Science of a Lost Art* (Pranayama, Vi Sama Vritti and extending the exhales)

BV - #0074 - 260421 - C103 - 297/210/7 - PB - 9781527280076 - Matt Lamination